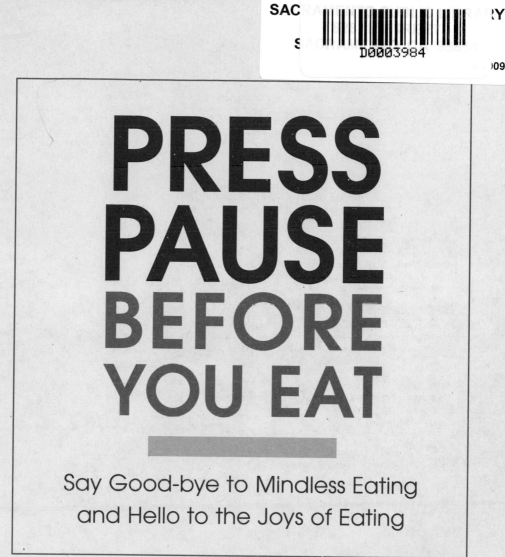

PRESS PAUSE BEFORE YOU EAT

Say Good-bye to Mindless Eating
and Hello to the Joys of Eating

LINDA MINTLE, PhD

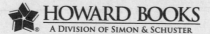

HOWARD BOOKS
A Division of Simon & Schuster

NEW YORK LONDON TORONTO SYDNEY

Our purpose at Howard Books is to:
- *Increase faith* in the hearts of growing Christians
- *Inspire holiness* in the lives of believers
- *Instill hope* in the hearts of struggling people everywhere

Because He's coming again!

HOWARD BOOKS
A DIVISION OF SIMON & SCHUSTER

Published by Howard Books, a division of Simon & Schuster, Inc.
1230 Avenue of the Americas, New York, NY 10020
www.howardpublishing.com

Press Pause Before You Eat © 2009 Linda Mintle

All rights reserved, including the right to reproduce this book or portions thereof in any form whatsoever. For information, address Howard Subsidiary Rights Department, 1230 Avenue of the Americas, New York, NY 10020.

Library of Congress Cataloging-in-Publication Data

Mintle, Linda.
    Press pause before you eat : say good-bye to mindless eating and hello to
the joys of eating / Linda Mintle.
        p.   cm.
1. Eating disorders—Psychological aspects.   2. Food—Psychological aspects.
3. Food habits.   I. Title.
    RC552.E18M554   2009
    616.85'2608—dc22   2008054185

ISBN-13: 978-1-4391-4864-8
ISBN-10:   1-4391-4864-3

10 9 8 7 6 5 4 3 2 1

HOWARD and colophon are registered trademarks of Simon & Schuster, Inc.

Manufactured in the United States of America

For information regarding special discounts for bulk purchases, -
please contact: Simon & Schuster Special Sales at
1-866-506-1949 or business@simonandschuster.com.

The Simon & Schuster Speakers Bureau can bring authors to your live event.
For more information or to book an event contact the Simon & Schuster Speakers
Bureau at 866-248-3049 or visit our website at www.simonspeakers.com.

Edited by Cindy Lambert
Interior design by Jaime Putorti

Scripture quotations not otherwise marked are taken from the *Holy Bible, New International Version*®, Copyright © 1973, 1978, 1984 by International Bible Society. Used by permission of Zondervan. All rights reserved. Scripture quotations marked MSG are taken from *The Message*. Copyright © 1993, 1994, 1995, 1996, 2000, 2001, 2002. Used by permission of NavPress Publishing Group. All rights reserved. Scripture quotations marked NASB are taken from the *New American Standard Bible*®. Copyright © 1960, 1962, 1963, 1968, 1971, 1972, 1973, 1975, 1977, 1995 by The Lockman Foundation. Used by permission. www.lockman.org.

To everyone who ever said, "Why did I just eat that?"
It's time to lose the guilt, become intentional, and enjoy eating!

CONTENTS

PART ONE
PURPOSE

1 Press Pause: It Takes Only a Moment   3
2 Hurry Up to Slow Down   10
3 Listen to Your Body Talk   26
4 From Impulsive to Thoughtful   43

PART TWO
ATTEND

5 The Many Meanings of Food   59
6 Relax and Put Down the Fork   75
7 Look Around: Hidden Cues That Make Us Eat   96
8 Food, Marriage, and Family   107

PART THREE
UNDERSTAND

9 Feasting on Emotions   121
10 The Power of Food Thoughts   142
11 Spiritual Hunger Requires Spiritual Food   163

PART FOUR

STRATEGIZE

12 Tackle Your Emotions 177
13 Renew Your Mind 200
14 Eating with People, Not Because of Them 212

PART FIVE

EXECUTE

15 Press Pause as a Lifetime Practice 229

Acknowledgments 233
Notes 235

PART ONE

PURPOSE

Pressing *pause* begins with purpose. To purpose to do something means to set out to attain a goal, to be determined to make something happen, to reach a decision or achieve a specific end. When we approach something with purpose, we become intentional about it. And that is exactly what we want to do with eating—become intentional about it.

While one of the purposes of eating is to provide the body with energy and nutrition, we also want to include the goal of eating with enjoyment. My intent is to help you transform the way you approach food and eating through the use of intention.

So let's begin with an intentional pause. We stop a moment and think about what we are about to do when it comes to putting food in our mouths.

This first section will equip you with three techniques to get started:

1. Purpose to slow down.
2. Purpose to listen to your body.
3. Purpose to be thoughtful.

As we slow down, listen, and delay a moment, we create a space to think, feel, and behave in new ways. When we do these three things, our journey toward intentional eating begins. Let's get started!

1

PRESS PAUSE:
IT TAKES ONLY A MOMENT

Suzy and I took our usual places in the overstuffed chairs in our favorite coffee shop. As we sipped our tall, skinny, one-pump decaf mochas, her eyes kept wandering to the display case of pastries. She seemed unusually distracted. "Suzy, I know my problem with the rabbits eating my begonias is not exactly front-page news, but you seem distracted. Is everything okay?"

"Huh? Oh, yeah, I guess so. I was just looking at those pastries in the display case. They look so tempting. I would really like an apple fritter with my coffee. My mouth is watering just thinking about it, but I know I shouldn't eat it. I've got to lose ten pounds. Oh, what the heck, I'm going to get it. It looks yummy. Coffee and pastry are great together."

Suzy headed for the counter, bought the pastry, and began munching on it while I resumed our conversation: "Here's what a friend of mine suggests for my rabbit problem. Whenever you have your hair cut, you should ask for the clippings and then spread them around the bed of the begonias. Supposedly, this keeps the varmints away. Sounds a little creepy to me. Like a *CSI* episode for furry critters . . . Okay, you're not laughing. What is up with you?"

"I just ate that apple fritter."

"I know. I was sitting right here, remember? I witnessed the crime."

"It's not funny. I do this all the time. I eat when I'm not hungry, and that makes me crazy."

"Well, then, stop it."

"If I could stop, don't you think I would have by now?"

"I suppose so. I'm sorry. I didn't mean to be insensitive."

"It's like I don't have control over this and then I end up gaining five pounds. It is depressing. I'm caught in this vicious cycle. I try to resist but have no willpower. Then I feel bad and could kick myself. So I try to be good, but then a pastry starts calling my name. And you know me. If it's calling my name, I'm going to answer!"

"Do you have to answer by eating it?"

"Yes. Otherwise, it wouldn't be a problem, right?"

"Wrong. Anytime you think there is only one choice, you create a problem. There are other ways to handle this. You have more control than you think you do. Look, I saw that apple fritter, too. It looked delicious and I thought about how great it would taste with my coffee. I wanted it just as badly as you did. But I've learned a little secret that really helps me when it comes to eating. I've learned to *press pause*."

"*Press pause?* What are you talking about?"

"I've learned to press a mental pause button and become more aware of my eating. Basically, I've learned to be more intentional with my eating. It doesn't mean I am perfect when it comes to food, but it sure has made a difference."

Press pause is more than a strategy. It is a mindset that has been the foundation of my work with clients in therapy and clinical practice for more than twenty-five years. As an eating disorders specialist employed by medical schools, hospital programs, public schools, universities, and private practices, I have used this technique to help people from all walks of life who struggle with food and eating.

My professional life has focused on developing strategies that work when it comes to food and living a healthy lifestyle. During the past six years, I have had the privilege to talk to an even larger audience through speaking, writing, and appearing as Dr. Linda on ABC Family's *Living the Life* television show. I often remind our viewers that you don't need to be in therapy to have issues with food!

In fact, have you ever said to yourself, *Why did I just eat that? I wasn't hungry. I can't believe I just ate that?* This book is for you and the rest of us who eat when we aren't hungry, eat without thinking, or overeat when we are full, then find ourselves saying, *I hate myself right now. What is wrong with me?*

Once we eat to our own regret, then our sense of defeat only leads to more overeating. What a vicious cycle! We don't want to overeat but do. Then we feel terrible, make self-disparaging remarks or excuse our behavior, feel even worse, and overeat more. We give up and give in. We tell ourselves that the food is more powerful than we are and that we can't defeat this inner urge or impulse. We are left feeling hopeless.

And statistics seem to bear us out. Despite the billions of dollars spent on diets and fitness products, Americans experience record rates of obesity and remain extremely weight conscious. According to a study in *The New England Journal of Medicine*, 90 to 95 percent of people who diet are unsuccessful in the long term[1]—and other studies indicate that most of those dieters regain their lost weight within one to five years![2] These are not encouraging statistics—just thinking about them makes you want to grab the hot buttered popcorn.

To make matters worse, after we eat something we don't really want or need, we don't usually tell ourselves to let it go and move on. Instead, we give in to the hopelessness of the moment. What we need to do is *learn from the moment:* think about *why* we just did what we didn't want to do and focus our efforts on changing this practiced habit rather than simply feeling bad about it or excusing it.

Let's be honest. We know the facts about food. I mean, look around you. We are saturated with information. We are bombarded by diet and fitness trivia. You can hardly pick up a magazine without finding recipes or reading about a new ab reducer. Truth is, these days you don't have to be a registered dietitian to make good food decisions!

Most overeating or unhealthy eating is not cured by more seminars on *what* to eat, another new and improved diet, or more creative exercise ideas. The problem most of us have is that we don't *do* what we know is good to do! What we need to focus on is *Why?* What is missing? Why do we eat when we aren't hungry?

Our lives are busy. Food is always available and oftentimes we eat without thinking. We need to *press pause.* Our goal is to feel in control of the food we choose to eat, rather than the food controlling us.

We want eating to be an *intentional* behavior under our control. Wouldn't it feel great to be in control of the apple fritter rather than have the apple fritter controlling you? Wouldn't you like to look at a yummy pastry and make an intentional decision whether you are going to eat it or not? Or if you do choose to eat it, to not feel guilty afterward? It can be done!

To get there, we must understand that eating is more than a physical act that satisfies hunger. It is emotional, relational, environmental, and spiritual. We eat when we are hurried, stressed, and feeling all kinds of emotions: happy, sad, fearful, and more. Eating can distract us from uncomfortable feelings or connect us to memories of love. Food comforts us when we are lonely or rejected. It distracts us when we are angry and calms us when we feel stressed.

We eat when we fight with our spouse, feel sexually insecure, are stressed by the demands of elderly parents, try unsuccessfully to comfort a screaming toddler, are frustrated with work, and so on. Food gives us pleasure and a momentary break.

We eat because we can. Walking past the smoothie bar and seeing those machines foam up tropical concoctions moves us toward the counter. A cold winter night is warmed by a hot cup of peppermint mocha. The television advertisement of chocolate topping on rich vanilla ice cream is virtually telling us to march to the freezer. Our environment provides ample opportunities and cues to eat and provides inviting choices. We respond.

And finally, we eat to satisfy a spiritual hunger that can't be satisfied with food. There is a natural emptiness in all of us, a longing for something beyond ourselves that can't be met through the natural appetite—but hey, that doesn't stop us from trying! Even though in the long run, food doesn't satisfy those empty places or work to calm us down, sometimes it seems to fill emotional and spiritual emptiness. It provides a stop gap, but a very short one, and in its wake leaves us with guilt, pounds, and poor health.

Understanding that there are so many possible triggers to eating when we are not hungry, we now recognize that examining *why* we eat is essential for life success. What are the triggers and how can we react in new ways? Unless we become aware of *why* we eat and learn to *press pause* before putting food in our mouth, eating will continue to serve unintended purposes and weight-loss efforts will fail. But most important, the enjoyment of eating will be gone forever!

Food gives life. Somehow we've lost that perspective. Food has become our enemy. We obsess, overindulge, and wish we could just eat without giving so much thought to it. But we can't. Thinking about why we eat will help us. We have to become aware of what we are doing, take a deep breath, and make changes.

The purpose of this book is to help you rethink your relationship to food. My hope is that you will enjoy eating and learn to use food in positive, life-sustaining ways. To do so, you need to *press pause*, to take a moment and think about the meaning we've given food in our lives. If we are to change our negative relationship with food to a healthy one, we must become aware of how we think about food and use it in everyday life.

So what do we do? What is the cure for hurried and unintentional eating? How do we shift our thinking? It is not as difficult as you think, but does require honesty and *press pause* moments. We must be truthful to ourselves and develop an awareness of *why* we eat. Once we know ourselves better, we can consider our options, decide to make changes, and take action.

Think about anything you own that uses a remote control. One of the beautiful things about a remote is that it has a button on it marked *pause*, which allows you to stop the movie or TiVo. With the *pause* button, you have control and choice. You decide what to watch or what you will do next. The *pause* button allows you a moment to reflect, to not react impulsively, and to determine your next move. This is what we need to do when it comes to food: press a mental *pause* button that allows us to be more intentional about our next move. It just takes a moment.

This book will show you how to use that *pause* button: how to *press pause* before you eat, to be in control and develop a thoughtful approach to eating, and to think more about what you do and why you do it.

Our moment-by-moment choices determine our future. We need to make changes that lead to happiness and health.

The basic Press Pause Principle is this:

Purpose in your heart to pause.

Attend to the moment.

Understand why and what you do.

Strategize ways to make changes.

Execute new ways to think, feel, and act.

Each chapter will walk you through the process of being intentional. You will learn to *press pause*, take a deep breath, reflect for a moment, and choose your direction. That's the pattern to develop in order to change your relationship with food. And it takes only a moment—a pause. Because we are body, soul, and spirit, this book will address all three aspects of our being. Our bodies are greatly affected by our eating habits, but so are our soul and spirit. Consequently, we will learn how to engage all three aspects of our being when it comes to food and eating.

At the end of each chapter, you will find a variation of the Press Pause Principle that relates to the theme of that chapter. Each of these principles is part of an overall plan to develop a healthy lifelong positive relationship with food and eating. Pressing *pause* is the key to intentional eating. It requires only a moment but greatly affects our lives.

The Press Pause Principle will help you remember how to make small but important changes. It is a summary of the information presented in each chapter and a reminder of how to approach food and eating with intention.

As we learn to recognize our eating triggers and understand why they are so powerful in our lives, eating takes on new meaning. It becomes enjoyable, not filled with guilt and angst. Most of us have lost the joy of eating and need to find it once again or maybe experience it for the first time. Whether you are underweight, overweight, or at your ideal weight, learn to look beyond *what* you eat, to *why* you eat. *Press pause* and choose the path to success.

PAUSE FOR WISDOM
Eat your food with gladness,
and drink . . . with a joyful heart.
ECCLESIASTES 9:7

2

HURRY UP TO SLOW DOWN

What? The alarm didn't go off. I've got a 9:00 a.m. meeting and I'm not even showered. Okay, jump in the shower, get dressed. I can skip breakfast and grab some coffee on the way to the train. I can't miss that meeting.

I feel like a taxi driver. My kids are constantly on the go. My van is our second home. Eating happens on the run, whenever we can fit it in. Check out the crumbs between the seats and on the floor. It's a mess. I keep a stash of nutrition bars and juice boxes on hand. Every once in a while I think about eating more healthfully, but I don't have time.

My job is stressful. I really don't have time for lunch. Most days I just work through lunch and buy a snack from the vending machines to hold me over until dinner. By dinner, I'm starving and overeat.

The baby is crying; the three-year-old just colored on the wall; the five-year-old is constantly getting into things. I don't sit down for even two minutes during the day. Meals? I make them for the kids, but I'm too busy feeding them to eat. Usually, I pick a little here and there off their plates. With naps, baths, preparing food, and keeping the house organized, I don't have time to think about eating. I couldn't even tell you what I ate today.

It was all a blur. I just know that I'm gaining weight, which seems crazy given how busy I am.

Sound familiar? Welcome to everyday life! In our hurried society, we are literally starved for time. The cell phone rings, the BlackBerry beeps, the driver behind us honks when we don't jump fast enough at the traffic light. Technology moves us faster and forward.

We rush our kids to activities—soccer games, music lessons, tutoring. We sign up for classes on time management, set goals, and hire consultants to manage our businesses. Time is opportunity and money.

Our pace is full speed ahead. We are annoyed when the Internet connection moves slowly, when movies aren't filled with action, and when we can't click the remote fast enough. We've equated speed with progress.

Eating on the Run

Busy schedules translate into eating on the run or skipping meals altogether. Life is not only filled with multitasking and hurried moments but on-the-go consumption. Eating becomes a thing to do while doing other things. I call this task snacking—eating while doing something else. Grab that bag of chips and munch while you are driving to the bank or picking up the dry cleaning. You have too much to do to slow down enough to eat sensibly.

Skipping meals and eating snacks is now called flexi-eating, and it's all about busy lifestyles: mealtimes are flexible and must fit into your lifestyle.[1] Here's how one research firm describes the trend toward flexi-eating: "Routine meals at home or with the family are declining. While snacking and eating on-the-go have been noticeable trends for a few years, it is no longer just about rushing—a flexible attitude towards eating has become the norm and we may rush a lot of meals or skip them altogether . . ."[2]

In other words, our attitude toward eating is changing. Meals float with our schedules. Food is an all-day consumption, not tied to time or space. Eat when you can, whatever you can, and where it's convenient. With the exception of planned leisurely dinners with friends or family, eating is determined by our *individual* schedules and preferences.

Our hectic days determine when food will be scheduled into our lives. Yes, we get hungry but we don't always have time to eat. So we turn to snacking and "grazing"—very seldom on healthy foods—for most of the day, fitting in meals where and when we can.

Reid, a single dad with two teenage sons, rarely sees his kids during the week. They come and go so often that most meals are prepared individually, usually in the microwave. Once the food is cooked, each person heads to his room or the television.

It's like a twenty-four-hour self-serve restaurant, with little interaction among family members. Nutrition is questionable. Mealtimes vary according to each person's daily schedules. What bothers Reid is that everyone eats whatever he wants, usually by himself, and on his own timetable. Reid misses his family.

I cringe every time I see the dancers at my daughter's ballet studio dining on vending-machine food. Most of them have been dropped off from school, haven't eaten since lunch, and are starving. But their only food choices are vending-machine snacks, because no one had time to pack them a healthy snack to eat before dance class or during their break.

We say we don't have time to eat in the morning. But we wake up with empty stomachs, so our low blood sugar levels cause tiredness, poor performance, difficulty concentrating, and irritability. It's no surprise that studies say that we're more prone to have an accident, to do poorly in school, and to feel tired midmorning.[3]

But breakfast is the meal most sacrificed for the sake of time, though any of us could get up ten minutes earlier and cook a bowl of oatmeal with raisins or spread peanut butter on toast. We would have to readjust our schedules, value breakfast, and choose not to rush. Instead, we make choices that rush us and lead to irregular eating habits.

The Cost of Rushing

Here's the question to ask: *Is this good for us?*

> *Can we stop long enough to think about the nutrition we actually get from vending-machine snacks and fast-food runs?*
> *Does coffee on an empty stomach really energize us to do our best work?*
> *Do juice boxes and nutrition bars truly fuel our bodies?*
> *Do we even enjoy eating while multitasking?*
> *Do we eat more than usual when we finally sit down for a meal?*

Most of us know we need to make some changes. Research tells us that rushing and feeling dissatisfied with life go hand in hand. According to the Pew Research Center,[4] people who feel rushed are less likely to be satisfied with their free time, job, family life, housing, income, and overall standard of living. Researchers have found a connection between rising obesity levels in our culture and the mentality of wanting things immediately.

But knowing this doesn't slow us down. Instead, we keep going, eating on the run, and feeling starved for time. The end result is dissatisfaction. We have relationship difficulties, anger, stress, depression, anxiety, disconnection, and spiritual emptiness. Rushing takes a toll.

Metabolism is like a fire in a fireplace. The fire burns best when logs are placed on it at regular time intervals. Without regularly adding wood, the fire goes out, but if you dump a boatload of wood on a fire, it will smother the fire. The best way to burn a fire is to continually give it fuel and stoke it. Going long hours without eating slows our body's metabolism. Eating at regular times is fueling and stoking the metabolism fire. Flexi-eating doesn't do the job!

We need to slow down and think about our choices. If we can schedule a meal and not eat on the run, eating becomes relaxed and enjoyable rather than something to rush through. And the greatest benefit is that we won't eat as much because we will be satisfied.

Why We Hurry

One reason we rush around like chickens with our heads cut off is because we are *conditioned* to be in a hurry. We get cranky if the fast-food lane isn't fast enough. At some eating establishments, the pizza is free if it isn't served in the allotted time. And if we have to wait too long at our favorite restaurant for the bread basket to arrive, we become testy. Patience is *not* our virtue.

Yes, we feel a need for speed and our culture reinforces it. *The early bird gets the worm. Time is money. You snooze, you lose.* We are caught up, rushed, and not considering the impact of this conditioned impatience on our physical bodies, emotional lives, relationships, and spiritual growth.

Rushing creates stress. Stress elevates adrenaline and cortisol levels, which interfere with our immune systems. All our rushing can lead to increased blood pressure and angry, irritable, anxious feelings. We don't sleep well and we feel fatigued. Most of all, rushing prompts us to act before we think.

We rush because we don't want to deny ourselves anything that might feel good at the moment. We grab the doughnuts because we see them by the coffeepot. We indulge in gourmet drinks loaded with calories because we like the experience. We dive into the ice cream because we had a rough day and need something to comfort us (and because it tastes really, really good). But indulgence rarely leads to contentment. Instead, it usually feeds an appetite for more.

Mindful eating requires focusing on the present and the future. What you do *now* affects your *future*. Choices are important. That high-calorie drink might satisfy an immediate craving but the extra calories will cause a future consequence. And that's the problem with living in a *now* society. We don't think about how the moment affects our future.

Even when we do consider the moment, we don't think about it in a helpful way. We don't know how to stay present in the moment (I'll cover this in chapter 4). For now, just remember that enjoying the moment and thinking about future consequences are both important to mindful eating.

The Virtue of Patience

The opposite of rushing is waiting or being patient. Another word for *patience* is *long-suffering*, not a word you hear often. It means to be slow in avenging wrongs. Long-suffering is born out of love and is an active response to opposition.[5]

Where do we feel the opposition to slowing down? In our culture, which reinforces our hurried state. It feeds us messages to hurry up, move faster, and be impatient. However, patience is a virtue and a character trait we value as good. It is a sign of maturity that ultimately brings inner peace and quietness to our souls. In fact, long-suffering is an attribute of God and evidence of our relationship with him. When we invite God to influence who we are and how we behave, we begin to grow more patient.

Cultivating patience requires an attitude of submitting and receiving versus doing and getting. It is a surrender of your need to be right and a willingness to submit to the work of God in you. Without God, patience is difficult to develop. But patience is what quiets us, slows us down, and allows us to think through the consequences of living a rushed and hurried life. Patience allows us to stop eating unconsciously and to think about our actions.

Are you ready to stop the madness of rushed living and trade it for a little peace, connection, and inner content? I want to enjoy eating and not always feel like I'm rushing through it to the next thing. I want to taste my food, not inhale it. But doing this requires patience.

Patience requires us to listen, breathe, and be in touch with our inner thoughts and reactions. It means waiting for an outcome without becoming stressed or upset. The patient person can set boundaries in a crazy workplace. He can say, "I'll work as hard as I can to meet that deadline, but I'm going to take twenty minutes to eat and take care of myself. I will *press pause* to reenergize my body and brain. With food at a regularly scheduled time, I will function better and faster."

Because our culture doesn't value patience when it comes to eating, it is something you must commit to developing. The food industry doesn't make as much money if you sit long enough to do more than inhale your food. Anytime, anywhere, anything is their motto. You want it. You can have it—now! Breakfast is served all day in some restaurants, and fast-food chains promote the late-night "fourth meal." Time doesn't matter. Eating transcends time.

Patience does not come easily for me. Years ago, when traveling with a television crew to Latin America, I was nicknamed La Furiosa! You don't have to speak Spanish to understand the translation. Sadly I was the ugly American who exhibited the "time is money" mentality. And it was clear that I didn't understand the cultural significance of taking time with a meal and resting. I had much to learn.

Patience is an active response that requires us to wait without complaining. It is a mindset involving the way we look at something. When patient, we refuse the impulsive and the hurried.

To exercise patience before you eat means not impulsively responding to false hunger and environmental cues that encourage eating anytime and anywhere. While driving my car, I may see a billboard advertising a hot fudge sundae. I think, *That sundae would really taste good right now.* Patience tells me to *press pause* for a moment. If I'm hungry, a hot fudge sundae isn't the best choice—I need something more nutritious and satisfying. If I'm not hungry, then I must consider the consequences of having a high-calorie, high-fat snack. I can consider if something else sweet would satisfy me, such as an apple or a yogurt. When I am patient, I can question if I am hungry and need other food, or if I'm simply craving the dessert and how it would make me feel to eat it. I have a moment to at least think about my answer.

Let's take a look at one man's triumph over impatience. Mike liked to say that he was impatient by nature. After a heart attack at age forty-three, he decided to question his assumption. Working with a therapist, Mike came to realize that his impatience was learned through the generations. Growing up, when little Mike tried to fix something, Dad would pull the tool out of his hand and say, "Let me do that. It's taking too much time." His grandfather treated Mike's dad the same way.

Mike realized that his father and grandfather didn't value the learning process. They valued getting things done in a hurry. Saving time was more important than teaching Mike how to do things on his own, and now Mike was doing the same to his children and wife.

This insight helped Mike realize that his impatience was learned and could be unlearned. He could lower his irritability and lessen his stress by becoming more patient with his family. He could take the time to teach them how to do things so he could do less. And he could slow down enough to mentor his children.

Making these changes required Mike to shift his thinking about time. Time isn't wasted when it involves mentoring and teaching, because the outcomes are worth the time taken. *The same is true about eating*. Taking time for a meal has positive outcomes worth the effort.

You Can Slow Down

If you're thinking, *I know it's probably good for me to slow down and make time for regular meals, but it just can't be done given my lifestyle*, ask yourself, *Why not?* If you want to change, you can. You can slow down. But you have to be convinced that it is important.

Think about why you are so committed to rushing around when hurried living is so bad for your health and mental health. Why are you so pressed for time? Why can't you slow down?

Slowing down is doable if you are committed to it. If you try to force yourself to change without the commitment, it won't last. Forcing yourself to slow down won't work unless you believe there is a real benefit.

You can find a thousand reasons why you can't slow down—and changing will be uncomfortable—but you can tolerate the discomfort and find a new way to live.

Slowing down in a culture that reinforces speeding up isn't easy, and change creates conflicts and anxious feelings. But pushing past those issues and having faith empowers us. We learn that we can do the healthy thing no matter how difficult it is.

Choose to Change: Bring Back Family Meals

One of the most difficult but rewarding changes you can make is to slow down your schedule and take time for family meals. Studies suggest that families who eat meals together

- ▶ decrease their child's likelihood to drink, smoke, or use illegal drugs[6]
- ▶ decrease their teen's likelihood to have sex at a young age, get into fights, be suspended from school, and be suicidal[7]
- ▶ improve nutrition and eat healthier foods[8]
- ▶ build relationships and intimate connections

▶ improve academic success in children, according to a study at the University of Michigan[9]

Is there something on this list that will motivate you to change from a flexi-eating pattern to scheduled meals enjoyed by all? Slowing down in a culture that reinforces speeding up isn't easy. But an intentional decision on your part, a commitment to slow down, will benefit your own health and the health of your family.

Reflect on the Toll of Rushing

Sarah, a single mom with three children, works outside the home while her kids are in school. She comes home for two hours and cleans the house, makes meals, helps with homework, and discusses the day with her children. Then she heads to a second job, and when she arrives home at 10:00 p.m., she checks on the kids and falls into bed. Some days, she eats only snacks all day. She is tired, out of sorts, and irritable. Her diet is severely lacking in nutrition.

Sarah knows she can't continue at this pace without consequences to her health and family life. And she is the only provider for her kids.

So she took a *press pause* moment and thought things through. She's slowly revamping her life. She's looking for a better-paying job that will allow her to give up her night job. She's reorganizing things around the house: her goal is to have breakfast and dinner with her family. She decided she can cook on weekends and freeze meals to thaw for weeknight dinners, and have her children help more with household chores.

Sarah has a plan and is choosing to change. She wants to live a less hectic life and be there to watch her children grow up.

Make Mealtime a Priority

Mealtime may be the one time during your day that you become quiet and centered. You can actually think about what you are eating and pay attention to internal signs of hunger—both help with portion control. But most of all, you have stopped the rush. You've created a *press pause* moment that will benefit your life.

If you live in a family, try to schedule meals together despite all the competing activity. If you commit to this change, you can make it happen.

In my family, mealtimes are different on different days, but are generally consistent from week to week. We eat dinner early on Mondays and late on Tuesdays because of soccer and ballet. On wacky Wednesdays, as I call them, half of us eat early and the other half eats later. If life gets crazy, this is the night we eat out. Thursdays we eat early and Fridays we eat around 6:00 p.m. The point is that we eat together as a family as many times as possible and try to have a relaxed time at the dinner table. We've decided that mealtimes are opportunities to connect with one another, to be relaxed, and not discuss the problems of the day or homework.

And here's a novel idea. Use mealtimes to talk about what you actually like about family members or friends and bosses. Use this time to encourage one another.

Because both my husband and I work outside the home, having meals as a family means we have to be organized, share domestic duties, and be creative. Mostly we have to plan ahead. We have many fast, fresh food recipes that can be whipped up in twenty to thirty minutes. You can find them online, in magazines, and on television cooking shows. Keep ingredients on hand so you can prepare a healthy meal in no time. Make a grocery list based on your favorite recipes, and on one regular night of the week, pull out your list, make a trip to the grocery store, and have everything ready to go.

I've dusted off my old slow cooker and put it into action. It's amazing what you can cook in that giant pot! And there is nothing like walking into the house after a long, stressful day welcomed by the smell of a delicious soup or stew cooking.

Sometimes I cook on the weekends and freeze meals for the busiest days. I make a big pot of chili and freeze it in meal portions for several meals. Or I might bake several banana bread loaves for breakfast and freeze those for hurried mornings. Cooking in bulk and freezing sauces and meals saves a lot of time and allows your family to eat together and have a nutritious meal. You will be less tempted to run to the fast-food drive-through when you know a thawed homemade meal is just minutes away.

All of this planning takes a little more effort but it's doable. We do it because we are convinced of the benefits. This is important to our well-being and that of our family. It is possible to make time for meals if you commit to it. If not, you'll continue to eat on the run, whenever, wherever, and whatever you can. And if you do, you and your family will pay a price.

When You Eat Out

Naturally, I'm not saying to never again eat out or walk into a fast-food restaurant. Reality check! We eat out. My family doesn't eat every meal together. We have teenagers! Our goal is to reduce the rushing, improve the quality of what we eat, and eat together as often as possible. Sometimes this means eating out. When we do, we try to make informed choices. Basically, we want to eat smart! Just remember that if you *press pause* and think about where you eat and what your options are, it helps. Here are a few general guidelines to consider when eating out:

- ▶ Choose a restaurant that offers fresh food—think deli style, salads, and fruit side dishes.

▶ Consider a grocery store for lunch instead of a fast-food stop. Many grocery stores offer fresh food entrées, with everything from homemade soups to freshly made sushi.

▶ Drink water instead of sodas.

▶ Order poached, grilled, or broiled.

▶ Watch portions; order the appetizer instead of the full entrée or share an entrée.

▶ Skip buffets and the endless bread basket.

▶ Skip dessert or share it with people at your table.

How to Slow Down

If you are still on the fence about patience, maybe this will help. *Impatience can make you fat!* Did that get your attention? Here's what researchers found. There is an interesting connection between the rising obesity levels we are seeing today in our culture and the mentality of wanting things NOW.[10]

Impatience says, *If it's in front of me, I'm going to eat it. Self-control is out the window.*

Patience says, *There are future consequences to think about. My choices are important. I have to slow down enough to think about what I am doing and tune in to my body when it comes to eating.*

Patience requires us to stop moving through life eating without thinking—to quiet our mind, to fill our spirit, to give up unconscious living and mindless choices. So how do you develop patience when it comes to mealtimes and eating?

Commit to the idea of slowing down. Refuse to think that you can't make changes because your life is too busy. Basically, dump all your excuses. You can make changes if you *want to do so.* Slowing down is a willful act based on the belief that this is important.

Imagine your life without all the rushing. What does it look like? What is different and what needs to change? Is hurrying through meals accomplishing your goals of eating well and enjoying food? Does it help stabilize your weight?

Create an eating space that is inviting. Let's lose the idea of eating while doing, and elevate eating to an act of self-care and enjoyment. Designate a place to eat. Make it relaxing and free from clutter.

Take time for meals. Restrain from eating whenever you feel like it. Develop a new perspective. Hurried lives aren't necessarily happy lives. Eating on the go has to stop or at least be minimized. Schedule meals and take time for them. Do what you can to plan ahead and make mealtimes less rushed. Allow yourself the time to connect with your family and your inner self. Make people, not time, your priority.

Stay humble. Life doesn't always revolve around you and your schedule. Is what you have to do so important that you should risk your physical and mental health? Stop running yourself ragged. Consider the consequences of stressful living. Model for those you love a better way to live. Do you have to answer your phone at the dinner table? Do you need to be on your BlackBerry while having a cup of coffee? There was a time when none of this happened and people actually got things done and enjoyed dinner and coffee.

Look inside. Why are you so impatient? This is important. Don't just say, "That's the way I am." Look at the reasons behind your impatience. Is it because you are inflexible, hold unrealistic expectations of others, believe you can control people, or lack compassion? Get to the root of your impatience. Once you know the *why*, commit to change. If you want to be calmer, then stop and embrace flexibility, become more realistic and compassionate, and learn to surrender control. Accept the moment for what it is—a moment!

Practice restraint. Don't get worked up over an extra five minutes in the grocery-store line. Take a moment to be kind to someone in line.

Adjust your expectations. Don't make a scene because someone didn't jump fast enough for your liking. Determine not to eat whatever is in front of you. Ask God to help you practice what isn't natural. Put on patience by inviting God to work in your life. Surrender to him and allow maturity to develop.

As you *press pause* concerning your hurried life, ask yourself these questions:

1. What would keep me from slowing down?
2. What would help me slow down?
3. What has helped me slow down in the past?
4. What benefits would I see?

Once you *believe* that slowing down and developing patience are good ideas, commit to doing both. Get rid of your ambivalence. Change begins in the mind and heart. You can do it. We are only talking moments. Take the time.

THE PRESS PAUSE PRINCIPLE

Purpose to slow down.

Attend to the toll that rushing takes on your body, soul, and spirit.

Understand that you have been conditioned to rush and be in a hurry.

Strategize ways to be more patient.

Execute changes:
- ▷ Slow down.
- ▷ Plan for family meals.
- ▷ Make time to eat meals instead of eating anytime, anywhere, and anything.
- ▷ Eat out with intention.
- ▷ Refuse to multitask while eating.
- ▷ Seek God's strength to maintain your new commitment.

PAUSE FOR WISDOM

*No matter what looms ahead, if you can eat today,
enjoy the sunlight today, mix good cheer with friends today,
enjoy it and bless God for it. Do not look back on happiness—
or dream of it in the future. You are only sure of today;
do not let yourself be cheated out of it.*

HENRY WARD BEECHER

3

LISTEN TO YOUR BODY TALK

Babies have an innate sense of knowing when they need food and when they are full. Their relationship with food is simple. But as we grow and develop, our relationship with food becomes more complex. That innate sense of knowing when to eat is often overridden by external signals that drive our appetite. Because of a host of environmental and social factors, we don't always eat when hungry and stop when full.

Think about all the times you've said, "I really shouldn't eat that because I'm full," but you ate it anyway. The other day, after eating half of a huge Greek salad, I was full. But when my son ordered an enormous piece of cheesecake for dessert, several forks accompanied it.

Before the dessert's arrival, my body was telling me to stop eating. But I ignored the physical signals. The cheesecake was so appealing: juicy, plump strawberries surrounded by chocolate drizzle and whipped cream had our mouths watering. Just the sight of food can stimulate appetite. It fires neurons in the brain and our bodies say, *Hey, I want more of that.* The sight of food can override feeling full.

But all it took was a few bites to quell the craving, and because I was mindful about what I was doing, I was able to put down the fork. No guilt, just the enjoyment of a sweet sensation.

If taste and sight aren't enough to kick up appetite, the smell of food can make us want to eat as well. Research says that smell prompts the secretion of insulin and makes us think we are hungry, explains Sharron Dalton, PhD, RD, in her book *Our Overweight Children*.[1] So the next time you pass the cinnamon buns baking in the mall, *press pause* and walk away. Give yourself a few minutes for the smell to dissipate and that urge to eat will pass.

The Temptation of the Forbidden

Appetite is also influenced by our diet-conscious culture that teaches us to ignore our bodies' physical sensations of hunger. We are given

Other Things That Influence Appetite

The sensory cues of the sight, taste, and smell of food are not the only factors that affect the desire to eat. Appetite is also influenced by temperature. Next time you walk into a restaurant, pay attention to the room temperature. We tend to eat more when the temperature is colder. Our metabolism drops and eating warms us up.[2]

It's also true that sipping ice water burns more calories because it temporarily raises our metabolism in order to keep our body temperature from falling.[3] So while you are ordering appetizers, ask for ice water instead of alcohol! Alcohol leads to overeating because it makes us feel less inhibited and impairs our judgment. This results in eating more because we aren't paying attention to our body cues or we simply don't care what our body is telling us.

the message to ignore hunger cues. *Deprive yourself. Don't give in. Suppress that appetite.* In this way, eating is associated with deprivation. Certain foods are off limits. Self-imposed restrictions apply. But in the long run, deprivation just makes us want something even more. Always thinking about how to resist food makes it even more desirable. Eating is reduced to a power struggle between our will and the temptation. Tell me I can't have that piece of cheesecake and I will want it all the more.

Personally I am tired of thinking about eating as another temptation. I want to look at food the way God originally intended—as pleasant to the eye and good to eat. I'd like to relax, be healthy, and put food in my mouth without feeling guilty. I don't want to be driven by diets, hurry, stress, emotions, impulses, or anything else that takes the joy out of celebrating a meal with others or enjoying a meal on my own. I want to eat a yummy chocolate and not regret it! I want food to be a *part* of my day, not the central focus.

To accomplish this, we must lose the idea of the forbidden. All food in moderation is the mantra of most dietitians. So let's stop thinking of food as something to always resist, off limits, or in the camp of good and evil. Instead, let's discover how to attend to our bodies and listen to what they tell us. To do so, we begin at an obvious beginning: learning to recognize physical hunger.

Recognize Physical Hunger

Hunger needs to become our primary cue to eat. But we have learned to ignore it, we don't recognize it when it hits, or we respond to environmental cues such as sight, temperature, and smell instead of internal cues.

When was the last time you were hungry, really hungry? If you are like me, it's been a while. I have two teenagers who claim to be in a constant state of physical hunger. "I'm starving" are the first words out of their mouths when they bolt through the back door of the house after school. They don't even notice me standing in the kitchen because their eyes are locked on the refrigerator like a radar target. Woe to me if I get in the way before they secure the target—food!

And your kids probably are hungry. Because school schedules have them eating at odd times, they grab snacks out of vending machines to ward off hunger until they arrive home. Their schedules don't allow them to tune into their bodies to determine hunger. When their bodies tell them they are hungry, they can't get to the food. So they learn to graze, eating whatever and whenever they can.

In my graduate school days, I could only afford those five-for-a-dollar macaroni-and-cheese boxes. And every bite of that high-carb goo calmed my growling stomach and kept me from biting off the head of anyone who dared cross me at that moment.

Now that I can afford to choose my food, I can have what I want, whenever I want it. Trust me, macaroni and cheese is not high on my wish list.

But just because we can choose from a variety of foods any time we want them doesn't mean we should indulge whenever we feel like it. Hunger needs to be our primary signal, or green light, to eat. This means we have to *press pause* long enough to focus on our bodies and recognize hunger. So when the hunger light goes off, sit at a yellow light for a few seconds until you decide to go or stop, and decide what to eat. When we pay attention to our internal cues, our bodies will tell us what to do.

An important question to ask is, *Do I recognize real hunger when it hits?* Many of us would say no. I asked a client who struggled with her weight to focus on what her body was telling her when she reached for food, to pause and ponder, *Am I really hungry?* Her answer, "I don't have to ask because it doesn't matter. My body says, 'Go ahead and eat' anytime I see food. Hunger has nothing to do with it."

But that wasn't her body talking. It was her mind and emotions. Deeply wounded by a recent betrayal, all she could focus on was escaping the anger and hurt inside. Her mind said, *Here's something that feels better than the emotional pain I feel: food. For the moment, it will take me away.* So when she drove past Krispy Kreme, walked through the candy aisle, or sat listlessly in front of the television screen, her emotional emptiness prompted her to reach for food. The pain of betrayal was not something she wanted to feel. Food was her escape. And it was pleasurable.

I pressed, "Would you recognize the physical signs of hunger if they were present?"

"Honestly, I don't think so. If I ate because I was hungry, I don't think I'd be sitting here with you."

True. If we ate only when we were hungry and stopped eating when we were full, I wouldn't be writing this book and you wouldn't be reading it! The truth is that we eat for all kinds of reasons, but hunger isn't high on our lists. And even if we are aware of being hungry, we don't always care or choose to pay attention to it.

For years, I ran groups for compulsive overeaters and learned much from those women and men. One thing I learned was that the signs of authentic hunger often had to be taught. Group members were generally not tuned into their bodies in terms of attending to the *physical* signals of hunger. Instead, they tuned into their emotions and ate in response to those feelings. Eating was a much easier path than dealing with personal anxiety.

Thus, we often began our group sessions with a reminder to tune into our physical bodies. What were they telling us? Are they our friends or enemies? Our goal was to cooperate with our bodies as friends and, aside from scheduled meals, to eat in response to true hunger, not as a reaction to an event, thought, or feeling.

Sounds simple, doesn't it? Well, it's not! We don't trust our bodies or listen to them, especially if we struggle with body acceptance. Our bodies feel like the enemy, always doing what we don't want them to do. So we fight food wars and diet until we can't take it any-more, never thinking of our bodies as useful or supportive of reaching our goals. Yet it's not our bodies that are at war. They signal us and tell us when we are hungry and full. The fight is really in our minds and hearts.

Physical hunger develops after hours of not eating and usually feels like this: a grumbling in your stomach and perhaps a slight pain or ache in your gut (that's why we call them hunger pangs). If you wait too long to eat, you may have a headache or light-headedness and experience irritability, a lack of concentration, and tiredness. Physical hunger usually builds gradually with a growing feeling of emptiness in the stomach. When physically hungry, you aren't usually picky about what to eat; you just want food.

Physical hunger differs from emotional hunger: it doesn't go away if you wait it out, while emotional hunger does. Physical hunger intensifies over time. Emotional hunger does not. Only the craving seems to intensify with emotional hunger. Physical hunger is relieved with food; emotional hunger is relieved through distraction or escape and avoidance, or, of course, through dealing with the underlying issues.

Identify Physical Hunger: Take the Hunger Test

Let's see how well you can determine if you are hungry. Close your eyes and focus on your body. Try to clear your mind of any thoughts or distractions. Assess where you are in terms of hunger now. Look for any of the physical sensations just described (growling stomach, headache, tiredness, and so forth). On a scale from 0 to 5, with 0 being very hungry and 5 being very full, rate your current state.

Once you've rated your hunger, think about when it was you last ate. How much time has passed since then? If it has been four or five hours since you last ate, you are probably hungry and experiencing some physical sensations—although for some people, physical hunger can build in a shorter time, particularly if they are eating lots of simple carbohydrates or if they are very active.

If you've recently eaten, you probably don't have those physical sensations. You may still want to eat, but not because you are truly hungry. The point is to tune into your physical body. What is it telling you?

You can practice this short exercise each time you are ready to eat. First, *press pause*, clear your head, close your eyes for a few seconds to minimize distractions, concentrate on the physical feelings inside your body, and rate your hunger on the 0 to 5 scale. If you are a 0, 1, or 2, you might need a small snack or a meal. If you are a 3 or above, try to delay eating until mealtime or when your hunger builds. This is a critical step in breaking unhealthy eating patterns.

Practically speaking, we can't always eat whenever we experience hunger. My kids can't eat their lunches during class at 10:30 a.m. What helps is regularly scheduling meals and snacks. Scheduled mealtimes help stave off hunger. If you ate breakfast at 7:00 a.m., you'd probably be hungry for lunch by noon. You may even be hungry for a small snack midmorning, because five hours without food usually creates hunger. Most of my dietitian friends recommend eating at regular meals and intervals to avoid that "starving" feeling that commonly leads to overeating. We experience a natural cycle of hunger and fullness when we eat at regular intervals. This cycle appears to be learned and tied to the clock.

But pay attention to whether or not you are actually hungry at the structured mealtime. If you aren't, you may want to eat later if possible, or just eat lightly and save a snack for later. Have structure, but still be flexible and listen to your body.

The Inner Workings of Hunger

Hunger is regulated by our digestive tract, hormones, and brain. Two biological groups are operating at the same time: one that stimulates appetite, and one that reduces appetite. When we are physically hungry, our stomachs empty and the hunger hormone ghrelin is produced in our gut. It drives our appetite and signals our brain that it is time to eat. As mentioned before, our senses can also stimulate appetite.

When we eat, the stomach and intestines stretch, which activates nerves in the stomach and upper intestines that tell our brain that we are getting full. A peptide hormone also tells the brain that we are full, and two other hormones cement the deal by telling the stomach to stop eating. It's then time for digestion.[4]

Leptin, a hormone produced in our body fat, also signals the brain when we are full. The more body fat we have, the more leptin we usually produce. It would seem to follow, then, that the more we weigh, the less hungry we become. Not so. As an article in the *International Journal of Obesity*[5] explains, it appears that as one's weight climbs to obesity levels, it is possible to become resistant to leptin.

It Takes Only a Few Bites

Linda Bacon, PhD, professor of nutrition, City College of San Francisco, believes that it takes only a few bites of food to enjoy it, because your taste buds lose their sensitivity to the chemicals in the food that appeals to you.[6] So if you can take the time to really enjoy just a few bites of your favorite dessert or snack, you will probably feel satisfied and not have to eat the entire serving.

Try a little experiment and see if it is true. Take your favorite treat and remove all the distractions around you. Then slowly take a bite, concentrate on how good it tastes, and enjoy the sensations of eating that bite. See if by the third or fourth bite you have been satisfied. You might be surprised!

So even though leptin's job is to tell the brain we are full, the message doesn't always get through.

The biology of hunger is complicated, involving multiple body systems, parts of the brain, the gut, and hormones. Suffice it to say that the brain and gut are busy balancing hormones that increase and decrease appetite and satisfaction. One group gives us the green light to eat; and the other, the red light to stop eating.

The key is to pay attention to the sensations your body feels when you come to a meal hungry and remember that it takes time for the brain to register that the stomach is full. The slower you eat, the more your body has a chance to register *full* and put the red light on eating.

Developing an awareness of hunger feelings is necessary to having a healthy relationship with food. Don't ignore those feelings. Trust your body. It needs to be refueled. Hunger is a signal telling us we need food. And if we wait too long to eat, we become ravenous and overeat or make unhealthy food choices. Our goal is to recognize the signs of hunger and not confuse them with emotional eating and other environmental triggers associated with appetite and hunger.

Liquids Fill You Out—Not Up!

When liquid diets were all the rage, I worked with a hospital that medically supervised a specific liquid diet. My job was to follow these patients behaviorally and help them comply with the diet. I noticed people were always hungry while on the liquid diet. They did lose weight but a year or two after the program, most of them had gained their weight back. They hadn't learned how to eat healthily and to listen to their appetite.

According to research at Purdue University,[7] liquid calories just don't give us those feelings of fullness we need to prevent overeating. So forget drinking your calories. Next time you are presented with the choice to have a fruit smoothie or an apple, *press pause* and reach for the apple. You will feel fuller.

Purdue University research also shows that drinking calories doesn't result in eating less. People who drank calories tended to overeat later in the day. Apparently, our bodies just don't register liquid calories the same way as solid ones.

So if you drink a protein shake in the morning for breakfast, chances are you will eat more during the day than if you began the day with eggs and turkey bacon or oatmeal and yogurt. This doesn't mean you should never have a delicious fruit smoothie. It means you'll need to pay attention to your food intake to avoid overeating the rest of the day.

Help Yourself Feel Satisfied

Three factors help make a food satisfying: weight, protein, and fiber. Researchers at the University of Sydney tested thirty-eight foods, and the most satisfying foods included whole-wheat bread, cheese, eggs, brown pasta (such as whole wheat), popcorn, all-bran cereal, grapes, porridge (such as oatmeal), baked beans, apples, beefsteak, ling fish (a type of cod), and oranges.[8]

Foods that scored low in terms of fullness and led people to overeat were those with lots of fat, sugar, and/or refined carbohydrates, including potato chips, candy bars, and white bread.

When we consider hunger, appetite, and satiety, we must listen to our bodies. Here are practical ways to work with all three:

Consider a small sweet at the end of your meal. Denying yourself will probably end in overeating later. And if you crave a sweet and keep eating other foods, you won't be satisfied. Better to eat a small sweet, such as a piece of fruit or one ounce of dark chocolate, to satisfy the craving.

Count the calories you drink. Remember, liquid calories don't make us feel as full as calories from solid food. With smoothies, coffee drinks, and other liquid confections, we can add many calories to our diet and still feel hungry.

Eat plenty of fiber, whole grains, fruits, and vegetables. They help you feel full, and have plenty of health benefits as well. All calories are not alike in terms of feeling full and warding off hunger.

Eat slowly so your brain can catch up. Remember it takes the brain around twenty minutes to register fullness. So take your time and enjoy what you're eating!

Schedule meals and snacks. Eat regularly—this will help you avoid overeating because you feel starved or famished.

Eat what you want—in moderation. Eat what you enjoy in reasonable portions that won't lead to weight gain. Ten rice cakes leave me unsatisfied and don't give me much pleasure. Better to eat reasonable amounts of a food you enjoy—such as a few nuts or a slice of whole-grain toast with a smear of jam.

Avoid emotional eating. Whenever possible, eat in response to physical hunger signs and not emotional hunger. Review the differences. You will learn new ways to respond to emotional eating in chapter 12.

Put it away. Out of sight, out of mind. If you don't want your appetite stimulated by the sight of certain foods, put them away in your freezer or cupboard, or walk away from the display case. Preferably, don't stock your home with foods that trigger you to eat when you are not hungry.

Use your remote. The sight of food stimulates appetite, so when food commercials come on television, switch the channel.

Have a snack or meal before grocery shopping. Shop when you are not hungry. We all tend to buy tempting impulse items when shopping hungry.

Use smaller dishes. The very presence of a large portion will prompt you to overeat and override your full feeling. You'll be more satisfied by the sight of a full small plate than a huge plate with a lonely but reasonable-sized serving of food.

Build satisfying meals. Meals containing protein, complex carbohydrates, fat, and fiber add to fullness. Pay attention to the composition of your meals. For example, include complex carbohydrates such as spinach, multigrain bread, lentils, and carrots, instead of simple carbohydrates such as white pasta or baked goods made with white flour.

Choose water. Drink water with your meals and between meals—no point in using up calories on beverages (soda, for example) that don't fill you up or give you much nutrition!

Start with soup. Begin a meal with a bowl of healthy soup including plenty of vegetables to add fullness. (A cream- or cheese-laden soup won't help with calorie control!) If you struggle with portion control and overeating, filling up on a bowl of soup before a meal helps.

Stay warm. Put on a sweater so the cold doesn't prompt you to eat more. Or become aware of the tendency to eat more when you feel cold.

Consider Your Shape

During one of our *Living the Life* television shows, the hosts and I discussed what works best in terms of eating and losing weight. What became apparent was that when it comes to losing weight, one size does not fit all.

Our bodies are different. Some of us burn calories faster than others, depending on our genetic predisposition and age. I know that seems unfair, but it is a factor you must consider in losing and maintaining weight.

And because our bodies are different, they respond to different eating plans and foods. So what works for one person may not work for another. From eating a high-protein, low-carb diet, for instance, my husband developed gout, a form of arthritis brought on by elevated levels of uric acid. He does much better on a diet filled with fruits, vegetables, yogurt, beans, and other healthy carbohydrates.

I, however, have a family history of diabetes, and feel best on a diet higher in protein and lower in carbohydrates. My husband and I have very different body chemistry and respond differently to foods.

We also have different body types. Research tells us that our body shape is a clue to how we gain weight and which foods work best for our bodies. A study by Dr. David Ludwig, director of the Optimal Weight for Life Clinic at Children's Hospital in Boston, found that round, apple-shaped people do best with diets that include fruits, vegetables, beans, nuts, whole grains, dairy products, and certain types of fat and that restrict simple carbohydrates such as white bread and white pasta. This is called a low-glycemic diet, and it stabilizes blood sugar better than high-glycemic diets. Low-glycemic diets are based on the Glycemic Index developed in the 1970s by Dr. David Jenkins. Basically, the index measures the carbohydrates in foods on a scale from 0 to 100, according to the amount that blood sugar rises after eating the food. The lower the score, the longer it takes that food to raise your blood sugar; this means that foods with lower scores ward off hunger longer.[9]

If you're apple shaped, you may do better on a low-glycemic diet, while low-fat diets may cause your blood sugar levels to fluctuate, making you hungrier. Check with your physician. It's worth experimenting with different foods to find out which ones work best with your body type.

Pay Attention to What You Eat

Try an intentional eating exercise that lets you tune into your body. First, place your meal on the dining table. Turn off the TV, radio, and computer. Take a few deep breaths and say a prayer of thankfulness for this food and the many blessings you have in life. Next, take a look at your food and appreciate what you see—the colors, the textures, the arrangement. Take a bite and chew slowly and concentrate on the taste. Stop between bites so you don't rush your meal. Monitor your thoughts. Are they wandering off to other things? If so, bring them back to the present. Attend to your body and stop eating when you feel full.

The point of this short exercise is to practice awareness of physical sensations in the body. By focusing our minds and concentrating on eating, we are much more aware of the physical sensations involved in eating. Tune into your body. It may be telling you more than you realize!

Manage Your Body's Insulin Production

When you produce too much insulin, you can feel hungry and gain weight. Insulin tells your body when you are hungry, it delivers food energy to where the body needs it, and it tells the body to save food energy by storing it as fat.

Because of the way we overload our bodies with carbohydrates and refined sugars, say Rachael and Richard Heller in their book *The Carbohydrate Addict's Diet*, we don't always absorb all the insulin our bodies produce. The excess ends up in our bloodstream, creating an imbalance that makes us crave more carbohydrates. Then we eat more carbs and produce more insulin. The end result: we gain weight and feel hungry.[10]

So it's important to eat foods that reduce your cravings. According to the Hellers, foods such as red meats, poultry, fish, cheese, tofu, oils, fats, dressings, nonstarchy vegetables (green beans, bell peppers, lettuce, asparagus, broccoli, and mushrooms) help reduce cravings.

The bottom line is to pay attention to your body. Which foods make you feel energetic? Which foods seem to stabilize your weight? Are you physically hungry, and can you recognize the signs?

Appetite, hunger, and satiety are complex subjects affected by biology and environment. Remember that your body gives you signals when it is hungry and full. You can *press pause* and learn to pay attention to those signals.

THE PRESS PAUSE PRINCIPLE

Purpose to tune in to your body.

Attend to what your body is saying. It's talking, so listen.

Understand the signs of physical hunger so you can distinguish them from emotional hunger.

Strategize ways to cooperate with your body as a friend and eat in response to recognized hunger.

Execute changes:
> ▷ Consider eating your calories rather than drinking them.
> ▷ Regularly schedule meals and snacks to prevent overeating.
> ▷ Use the practical tips in this chapter to help recognize and respond to appetite, hunger, and fullness.
> ▷ Notice your body type and (after having blood sugar levels checked) experiment with eating to stabilize insulin.
> ▷ Try a few bites of a food and see if you feel satisfied.

PAUSE FOR WISDOM

The body never lies. It's your spiritual tuning fork.
So it's your responsibility not to merely cover up its signals
with expensive lotions and Pepto-Bismol but to sit down
and really listen to what is underneath those symptoms.

SARA BEAK

4

FROM IMPULSIVE TO THOUGHTFUL

There it sits—beautiful in its tall glass and spilling over the sides. Mounds of creamy white vanilla bean ice cream topped with thick hot fudge sauce, fluffy whipped cream, and a round red cherry. You stare at it. You can taste it! You want it. But dessert will be served at the big dinner you are attending later. Should you save your calories for then or indulge now?

But everything in your body screams, *Go for it. Look how inviting it is.* You grab the spoon and shove the first bite into your mouth. All you can think about is the immediate pleasure that is about to hit your senses. Your impulses are controlling your behavior.

This scenario is repeated monthly, weekly, even daily for some of us. Regularly we are presented with tempting foods that tantalize our senses. Our decision to resist these foods or to give in and indulge is a complicated one.

We should be able to enjoy a beautiful ice cream sundae. Eating it is not "wrong" or bad. It is okay to enjoy the moment the spoon hits your mouth and you taste the flavors. But we don't want to act impulsively and eat things we really don't want or need—especially if we're going to regret it later. If we are eating only because the treat is in front of us and don't really want or enjoy it, that can be a problem. Eating impulsively can add unwanted pounds and bring guilt. Enjoying the moment doesn't mean losing control over your brain.

Do we forgo the treat or do we eat it? If we are always *now* focused and don't consider the future, we will struggle with eating. There are simply too many opportunities to eat when we aren't hungry and to indulge our senses. Giving in every time we have an opportunity is not mindful eating.

Find a Balance

We need to achieve a balance between gratifying ourselves and thinking about the impact of our actions. This requires a mental shift for most of us, because we live in a culture that values, encourages, and promotes immediate gratification. Yet successful living often requires the use of restraint over impulses.

Think about impulsive living on a broader scale than just eating. Many people spend money they can't afford, drink too much, take drugs, or gamble. We snap at people, yell at our kids, and silently fume at work.

Are we unaware of the future consequences? Have we never heard that smoking is associated with cancer or that stress hurts our bodies? Are we aware of the toll gambling takes on personal relationships and finances? Of course, but we aren't thinking ahead when we engage in these behaviors. Our choices are not informed by the consequences of our actions. When we act impulsively, our brains are given permission to take a brief vacation.

We make unwise choices in many areas of our lives because we are focused on the immediate benefit and ignore the future consequence. We simply choose not to think about the consequences. Our focus is only on the *now* and satisfying our appetites.

So the challenge is to enjoy the moment but not give in to the moment if it is motivated by an impulsive, mindless act. *Press pause* and decide if this food is something you really want to eat at this time. Give yourself thirty seconds to think before you act. Are you going to enjoy this and be sorry later?

Base your decision on your goals: to be more intentional, less impulsive, and more insightful about eating. Don't base your decision on pure sensation.

Good Intentions Don't Win the Battle

Information on how to eat well is easy to find. Everything from television shows to books to Web sites educates us about the role that good nutrition plays in our health and well-being. Most of us understand the basics. Food choices and portion size play a significant role in our health. Eating smart helps us feel good.

Yet with all this helpful information, we are not always eating smart. We are getting heavier and increasing our risk of disease and obesity-related health problems.

In our hearts we purpose to eat right, be fit, and feel good about our lives. But something happens that undermines our good intentions. Instead of making good choices, we reach for the high-fat, sugary, empty-calorie treat that doesn't help us reach our goals. We give in to immediate gratification.

So what happens between our good intentions and our actual behavior? A disconnect occurs. Our goal of eating well goes out the window in certain situations. Let's take a look at three situations that influence our choices:

- ▸ Being hungry and having too much time between meals or snacks
- ▸ Being busy
- ▸ Being away from home

When we are hungry, busy, and away from home, our food decisions are not based so much on what is good for us. Rather, we tend to make impulsive decisions that immediately gratify our need to eat. The busier our lives, the more we eat on the run and grab something out of hunger, the more likely we are to not attend to good food choices and portion control. Instead, we act on our need for immediate gratification. Information on health and disease takes a backseat to the pressing need of eating.[1]

Why We Give In to Our Impulses

We are presented with food temptation all day long on commercials, billboards, and advertisements. Food is ever present. And you can't simply remove yourself from tempting situations because food is so easily available. You don't have to go to a bar or score a hit in the alley to get food.

Reward yourself! Have it your way! You are the boss! You deserve a break today! If it feels good, do it! The messages to satisfy our desires are repeatedly pounded into our brains. The pull we feel to eat impulsively has nothing to do with being intentional; it is just the opposite. Advertisers want us to react, not think.

So it's easy to give in to the immediate. Advertisers count on us to be swayed by the images and slogans they present. The end goal is to get us to succumb to our impulses. The more we indulge, the more money they make. We are culturally positioned to be impulsive.

We also give in to eating when emotionally distressed. Emotional distress can undermine self-control. Our senses can rule our brains and shift the control from the long term to the present. When this happens, we give in to the immediate to satisfy our distress. This usually creates *more* distress when we regret having eaten impulsively.

We eat and overeat in response to not only emotional distress but to happy feelings as well. We are taught to celebrate with food and indulge when happy.

And just thinking about a food can influence us. According to Brian Wansink, PhD, in his book *Mindless Eating*, studies show that if we think about food and its tempting delights, we will probably eat it because our bodies respond to the thought.[2] They kick into gear, ready to receive the tasty treat. So if you are imagining a big gooey cookie with your latte, you will probably end up eating it. Visualizing the food and thinking how good it will taste will prompt you to be impulsive.

Add to this our biological makeup and it becomes even more difficult to resist impulsive eating. Just the sight, smell, or taste of a food can activate the parts of our brain associated with emotions. When we give in to immediate food rewards, emotional parts of our brain activate. These parts don't see the long-term consequences of a behavior and encourage us to satisfy the craving.

Developing Self-Control

If we want our actions to fit our intentions, we must develop self-control. Self-control requires us to delay the immediate and wait for the long-term reward. When it comes to food, this is not so easy for most of us.

Conversely, long-term decisions that require delay and thought are activated in parts of the brain associated with abstract reasoning, according to a study cited in the *Harvard Gazette* in 2004.[3] The emotional parts of our brain can win out over the reasoning parts when we know that an immediate decision will bring us reward. That's why we give in to the ice cream sundae. Different parts of our brain are competing with one another. The question is if the emotional parts that crave satisfaction will win over the reasoning parts that recognize long-term consequences. Yes, if you eat without intention. It takes intention to commit to the goal of learning to delay gratification. Giving in to the pleasure of eating just because we want the immediate sensation usually results in regret. Becoming mindful can prevent that.

One Marshmallow or Two?

Years ago a psychologist named Walter Mischel conducted a classic experiment to see how well four-year-old children could delay gratification. Fourteen years later, he looked at those same children to see what impact this ability to delay gratification had on their lives.

The experiment came to be known as the Marshmallow Test. Dr. Mischel put four-year-olds one by one in a room with a marshmallow and a bell. The kids were told that they could ring the bell and eat one marshmallow immediately or wait until the researcher returned in ten to fifteen minutes and get two marshmallows—that is, delay gratification and get a bigger reward.

Some of the children waited for the larger, delayed reward of two marshmallows. Others grabbed the one marshmallow the minute the researcher left the room.

The kids who waited engaged in various ways to distract themselves to restrain themselves from eating. They covered their eyes, made up games, sang, talked to themselves, looked around the room. Basically, they did everything they could think of to exercise self-control. What they didn't do was stare at the marshmallow and hope they could resist.

Fourteen years later, according to a report in *Developmental Psychology,* the kids who had waited so they could get two marshmallows turned out to be more academically successful; scored higher on their Scholastic Aptitude Tests (SATs); were more personally effective, self-assertive, trustworthy, dependable, and socially competent; and coped better with the frustrations of life.[4]

The Marshmallow Test highlights the need for impulse control. Our ability to delay gratification helps us live better lives.

And delaying gratification can be taught and practiced. We know from research cited by Roy F. Baumeister, Todd F. Heatherton, and Dianne M. Tice in their book *Losing Control,* that people who have trouble controlling their impulses are more prone to addictions, violence and crime, teen pregnancy, school problems, debt, and a host of other problems.[5]

All our lives we will be faced with decisions to give in to the immediate or wait for the long-term reward. Eating is only one arena where this life skill affects our happiness and goal achievement. So let's move beyond good intentions and start practicing the art of delaying gratification.

Ways to Delay Gratification

So what helps us learn to not be controlled by our impulses?

Eat more often. The first step is easy. Don't allow so much time between meals and snacks. The shorter the interval, the better you can plan food choices. The hungrier we feel, the more we allow our emotions to rule. We eat cookies or doughnuts instead of foods that will satisfy our hunger. Don't wait so long to eat that you make poor food choices. Typically, when you go more than four hours between meals, you forget about nutrition and reach for what is available, according to Lisa Mancino, PhD.[6] So keep the intervals reasonable.

Distract yourself. Learn a lesson from the four-year-old marshmallow eaters. Don't sit in front of the marshmallow and hope you can resist. Distract yourself. Resist the temptation by moving away from it. Think about what those four-year-olds did when they decided to wait for the two marshmallows. They sang, looked away, made up games, talked to themselves, and did whatever they could to distract themselves. You can do the same. When you *press pause* and determine that you don't want to eat a particular food, distract yourself. Leave the room, go for a walk, read a book, and do something to take your mind off the food.

Have a nibble. If you have difficulty delaying gratification when it comes to eating, have a snack. We give children small snacks to hold them over until mealtime, and you can do the same. Drinking water can also help, and limit simple carbohydrates such as chips, candies, cookies, sodas, refined breads, and cereals. These are more easily digested and absorbed, and cause a spike in blood sugar, which makes your pancreas pump out insulin. This leads to more hunger, sugar cravings, binge eating, and weight gain. Instead, reach for a snack of unrefined carbohydrates and protein, such as an apple and a slice of cheese, a slice of ham on whole-grain bread, or celery spread with peanut butter.

Plan ahead. Prepare meals in advance and keep healthy snacks on hand. This helps prevent impulsive, mindless eating. It does require you to think in advance about meals and go grocery shopping, but you will eat better and not as easily respond to the convenience of junk food.

Have an emergency plan. For those busy times, know where you can find healthier convenience foods. Think ahead in terms of where you can go to grab a fast bite that will help fill you up, satisfy you nutritionally, and be convenient. Some fast-food menus have a few healthy choices. Know those before hunger hits so you can make a good choice. Consider grocery-store salad bars. You can also phone in an order before your lunch break so that you don't have to wait for the food to be prepared.

Believe That Your Actions Matter

It is easy to feel that we are swimming upstream when it comes to fighting off the immediate. If we believe too much is working against us, we will struggle more with delaying gratification. Our beliefs matter.

If you have a strong belief that your actions can influence events, you have what psychologists call an *internal* locus of control. When it comes to eating, you believe you can delay gratification because your actions matter. Having an internal locus of control helps you stay on track because you believe that what you do matters.

People with an *external* locus of control believe that they have little control to delay and are at the mercy of external forces to determine their actions. They believe it doesn't matter what they do, because outside forces are working against them and will win in the end.

To delay impulsive eating, believe that your actions matter and focus on the goal. Have a vision of what you want to do with your eating. If you want to enjoy the moment, make good decisions that you won't later regret. Pause and decide: Do I want to eat based on impulse or do I really want to eat this? Make your mission one of thinking before you act.

The bottom line is that the better you can match your intentions with the way you actually eat, the less impulsive you will be and the better you can delay gratification. The key is to not allow factors such as increased hunger, busyness, and convenience to rule your choices—and to believe that self-control is possible.

Why Our Self-Control Lapses

Self-control has to do with restraining our emotions and impulses. It is our ability to control our passions and appetites. Self-control fails when our goals are in conflict. We want the immediate pleasure of

food but do not want to eat impulsively, and those goals are in opposition to each other. The tension must be resolved. Only we have the
power to choose which direction we will go.

The second reason our self-control often fails has to do with being mindless or unaware of our behavior. We react without thinking
and do not *press pause* to become aware of our behavior. Awareness
and self-examination are critical in living a good life. But self-control
also fails when we depend on our own willpower to make the right
choices. Self-control that is dependent on human strength to get us
through the moment is undependable. When our immediate desires
war with our long-term goals, our human strength often gives out.
We fail, feel miserable and discouraged.

About two thousand years ago, a man named Paul wrote of this
very struggle in the book of Romans. "What I don't understand
about myself is that I decide one way, but then I act another, doing
things I absolutely despise. . . . I realize that I don't have what it
takes. I can will it, but I can't *do* it. I decide to do good, but I don't
really do it; I decide not to do bad, but then I do it anyway. My decisions, such as they are, don't result in actions. Something has
gone wrong deep within me and gets the better of me every time"
(Romans 7:15–20 MSG).

Sound familiar? It seems like Paul has read my mind! And I find
it comforting that I am not alone in this struggle. Neither are you.
The fact is, this struggle with willpower is universal. Fortunately,
Paul doesn't leave us there. The fix is to tap into a strength source
bigger than ourselves in order to allow self-control to operate effectively. You see, attaining self-control over our appetites has little to
do with willpower and everything to do with a power greater than
ourselves.

The Source of Strength

Willpower is based on human strength. And while we may have moments of success using our human efforts to withstand temptation, in the long run, we usually fail. That is why so many dieters end up falling off the dieting wagon. They rely on their willpower to bring about change. Radical change takes something more, something that transcends our human nature to bring authentic discipline to our lives and sustain it.

That source is the power of God living in us. Because God chooses to have union with us, when we surrender our lives to him, we have his Spirit working inside of us, helping us to overcome temptation. As we yield control to God, his Spirit empowers us to do what we normally find difficult to do. Self-control becomes a byproduct of our relationship with God, not something that comes with self-denial or human mastery. God's Spirit in us influences our thoughts and emotions and gives us the power to exercise self-control.

Through this power, we can delay gratification and resist temptation. Augustine said it this way, "Sin comes when we take a perfectly natural desire or longing or ambition and try desperately to fulfill it without God. Not only is it sin, it is a perverse distortion of the image of the Creator in us. All these good things, and all our security are rightly found only and completely in him."[7]

If we apply what Augustine says to eating, we conclude that trying to handle our desires on our own and fulfill them without God is sin. Why? Because we are looking for fulfillment apart from God.

The temptation to indulge is perfectly natural. But if we give in every time, we have no discipline. And unrestrained indulgence doesn't bring ultimate fulfillment. But with the power of God working in us, we can withstand temptations and think about our behavior. We can make decisions to eat or not eat based on our awareness.

God's power is internal and doesn't come from willpower or our striving and effort. When we face food temptations, we always have the power to choose when the Spirit of God is in us. We may feel weak but his power is strong and helps us resist those things we choose to resist.

Self-control is possible when the Spirit of God is in you. Without him, we resort to willpower, which has a track record of low success. But with him, we may *press pause* and think before we act impulsively. True self-control comes through a relationship with God. His Spirit working in us empowers us and gives us the ability to be mindful, to delay gratification, and make choices with great freedom.

THE PRESS PAUSE PRINCIPLE

Purpose to delay immediate gratification.

Attend to the moment but also be mindful of the future. Both affect decision making. You want it now but will you regret eating it later? Attend to this thought.

Understand that good intentions and willpower don't win the impulsive battle. Too much is working against you—cultural pressure, biology, emotional distress, hunger, busyness, and convenience. True strength comes through a relationship with God.

Strategize ways to incorporate spiritual help. Invite God's Spirit to work within you and discover his strength to improve your self-control.

Execute changes:
> ▷ Shorten the intervals between meals.
> ▷ Limit simple carbohydrates (pasta, cakes, cookies, breads, sodas).
> ▷ Distract yourself.
> ▷ Eat a small healthy snack to stave off hunger.
> ▷ Plan ahead by preparing meals and knowing where you can find healthy convenience foods.
> ▷ Pray for strength and meditate on scripture.

PAUSE FOR WISDOM

One of the very nicest things about life
is the way we must regularly stop whatever we are doing
and devote our attention to eating.

LUCIANO PAVAROTTI, MY OWN STORY

PART TWO

ATTEND

Do you spend so much time thinking about the past or future that you can't relax and enjoy the moment? Regret that piece of cake and feel consumed by guilt, or deprive yourself because you want to be ten pounds thinner for an upcoming event?

Past guilt and longing for things to be different in the future can keep you from feeling joyful and alive in the present. In his book *Secrets in the Dark*, respected Christian author Frederick Buechner says, "Listen to your life. All moments are key moments."

Do we see all moments as key moments? Can we suspend our past guilt and discouragement and attend to now?

Intentional eating involves attending to the present moment. The moment provides us new opportunity to awaken to *now*. And when it comes to eating, we want to attend to the moment to increase our enjoyment of food. Attention brings the awareness necessary to better understand our relationship with food and eating. The moment can trigger unhealthy eating if we are unaware of it.

In this section, we will attend to the meanings we give food, our levels of stress, and the environmental cues that lead us to eat more than we intended. We will discover how to *press pause* and attend to our body, mind, and spirit. We will learn to create a space to think, feel, sense, and be.

5

THE MANY MEANINGS OF FOOD

I was shopping one day for a dog collar that would reflect the personality of my poodle, a loyal companion of many years. I didn't want your average pet-store collar—that seemed too ordinary for such a remarkable dog. So I thought I'd try a specialty pet store.

If you've never been to a high-end pet store, it's quite the experience. My first thought was, *I should live this well!* Beautifully displayed were gem-studded collars, designer sweaters, holiday costumes, soft luscious blankets, doghouses that looked more like Vegas hotel rooms, and a host of extravagant and pricey accessories.

As I slowly moved down the aisles, I spied the food display. A gourmet spread was laid out to tantalize the human imagination: multishaped biscuits dipped in something that resembled chocolate, rounded cookies with colorful sprinkles, carob truffles, peanut butter crunches, and fudge-like treats that looked like they deserved my best crystal platter. Even the names of these confections were inviting.

I was mesmerized. Wouldn't my precious companion *love* one of these doggy delights? How could I resist? As I began placing a variety of treats in my purple pet take-out bag, I paused and thought, *What am I doing? This is tempting but just wrong!* My dog doesn't know the difference between a dimestore biscuit and a three-dollar Bark for Joy bar. I was the one enamored of these mouthwatering delights. In my mind, giving my dog special treats meant giving her love, an association I had learned from childhood.

I flashed back to arriving home after Sunday church when I was a child and smelling the pot roast, potatoes, creamed vegetables, and homemade cherry pie. My mom worked a full-time job but was a wonderful cook and always had a great meal for us. And her sisters and in-laws tried to outdo each other in the baking department. Rich, warm strudels, fresh strawberry pies, thick fudgy brownies, and hot apple dumplings were just a few of the culinary treats we regularly sampled. And the motivation behind all the cooking and baking was love and affection for family. Food brought us together. It bonded us one to another. Today, just the smell of those foods evokes fond memories of family events and relationships.

Standing in the pet shop, I was responding to a similar association—food is love. The message was that if you loved your pet, you would be willing to spend a small fortune on delectable treats. The problem is that food is *not* love. It can be an expression of love, or even a part of love, but not love itself.

My family's love extends far beyond our regular dinners together. And my affection for my pet doesn't depend on gourmet goodies, especially since she doesn't know the difference. But we often connect food with love. And it has taken me a while to figure out that the two don't have to be bedfellows.

Food as Comfort

Think about it. When you needed comfort, did your mom bring you a plate of broccoli and say, "Here, honey. This will make you feel better. It's healthy and will strengthen your body." Not in my house! Security, comfort, and love were associated with warm fresh bread, homemade ice cream, and hot cocoa on winter nights. The association between food and love was woven into my DNA. Love me, cook for me. Love me, take me to dinner!

It's easy to pair food with love. And when we need love, we don't salivate for the vegetable platter. We want those comfort foods—mashed potatoes and gravy, ice cream, puddings, and cookies.

Our favorite love holiday is Valentine's Day. The more chocolate, the better! And when we want to show love to our precious pets, marketers count on us to make that association between love and food.

Whether we are aware of it or not, we ascribe meaning to food unrelated to its intended purposes. Food can mean love, comfort, companionship, and a host of other meanings. At times, we confuse what we *want* (love) with what we *need* (food). Eating to feel love and eating because you are loved are also very different.

So here's what I'd like you to do right now: *press pause* and jot down some ideas about what food means to you. See what comes to mind. Maybe you've never thought about what food means to you. That's okay too. This exercise will increase your awareness concerning the role that food plays in your life—the first step to change. How you think about food has everything to do with how you use it. If food means love, can you show love in other ways? Or will food be your only expression of love? If so, food becomes overly important as an expression of love.

If food is your friend, you won't give it up until you replace it with another friend. If food is a reward, you will have to identify other rewards, or you'll keep using food to reward yourself, which can be a problem if you're choosing unhealthy food or gain unwanted weight.

Once you figure out what food means or what needs it fills (more on that later), you can decide if you want to continue thinking about food in that same way. Or you can explore a new way to think about food—one that helps you eat joyfully and without guilt. And you can still give love, have friends, and get your needs met, too.

So what does food mean to you? Keep reading. Remember, our goal is to develop a healthy relationship with food and our minds. Here are a few ideas to get you started. Depending on your ethnicity, your family background, your experiences, and your culture, food will have specific meaning in your life. So *press pause* and ask, "What does food mean to me?"

Food and Culture

In most cultures, food is a way to connect with family and friends. It brings a sense of belonging. With my own European roots, mealtimes brought our extended family together. And what we ate was very influenced by the ethnic roots of our family.

My grandparents and father came from Germany and they were used to using grain, butter, and milk in most foods. In Germany grain was easy to grow and there was plenty of land for cattle. Beer was made out of barley, and butter comes from cow's milk. So milk, cheese, breads, and butter were staples of our diet. I never knew a vegetable that wasn't creamed or a meal without multiple starches.

Alcoholism ran in one side of my family, but my father made the choice to live a sober life. Even so, family get-togethers involved relatives drinking beer. But let me smell strudel baking in an oven, goulash cooking on the stove, or potato pancakes frying on the skillet and I am a happy woman. The smells evoke memories of festive family gatherings. Good food, good times, and good eating. We appreciated the cooks whose hands labored to prepare our meals and reveled in the eating. I enjoyed these home-cooked, unprocessed meals, and never had a weight problem when consuming them—probably because they were simply part of the experience, so I was content to eat only reasonable amounts.

As you think about your cultural roots, jot down some meanings of food. In many cultures, food means love, gathering, and connection. None of these are things we want to give up. But it is possible to have all those things, enjoy the meals, and not overeat. However, when food is the only way we receive love, community, and connection, we are in trouble. Food is one expression and others must be developed. Many of us have lost the ceremony and positive meanings associated with eating.

As a teenager, I would watch my grandmother preparing strudel, stretching the thin pastry sheets over the kitchen table and filling them with fruit. As she worked, she often told stories of her childhood and talked to me about her life. I was less focused on the food and more involved in the connection I was deepening with my grandmother. Although the pastry she prepared was high in fat and loaded with calories, I wasn't thinking about how many pieces I could have or that I should resist this dessert. This food was a part of our lives and history, like a familiar picture over the fireplace. It was a part of the scene, not the entire drama.

We want to connect with our cultural roots by choosing meaningful foods, preparing them, eating with full enjoyment, and celebrating together. Food and culture are good things. So think about how specific foods connect us to our historical roots and identities. This is positive and something to embrace, not deny. Eating these foods connects us to our roots—but we can eat them in moderation.

Food as Celebration

Have you ever planned a wedding or been involved in the planning of a wedding? One of the details includes the menu for the reception. Food was the last thing on my mind when I was planning my wedding! My fiancé and I were poor college students, so I would have happily settled for cake and punch at the reception. Simple, cheap, and easy—but not an option. In my family, you don't celebrate any-

Explore Your Cultural Roots

Food reminds us of our ethnic heritage and can link us to our ancestral past, reaffirming our historical identities. Food rituals and ceremonies such as the Passover seder meal are history lessons and tie us to previous generations.

Kwanzaa, an African-American holiday celebrated with family and friends, comes from a Swahili phrase meaning "first fruits of the harvest."[1] It focuses on traditional African values of family, community, responsibility, commerce, and self-improvement; it brings together communities to give thanks for accomplishments during the year. The celebration is joyous and includes singing, dancing, and of course food. Food recipes that pay tribute to African-American heritage are passed on from generation to generation. The menu might include black-eyed peas, greens, sweet potato pudding, corn bread, fruit cobbler, and other special family dishes.

Food is also very much a part of Hispanic culture. Whether it is used to celebrate Independence Day, Cinco de Mayo, or a birthday, families come together to eat special foods prepared for such occasions—such as the turkey, tamales, shrimp patties, romeritos, bacalao, and atoles of a Mexico City Christmas. Caramels and other treats kick off the holiday eating on the Day of the Virgin of the Immaculate Conception in Nicaragua.

As in many cultures, Hispanic foods vary from group to group, region to region, and country to country. If you come from Cuba, Southern Mexico, Central America, or Venezuela, you would use black beans. Dominicans and Puerto Ricans use pintos or pinto beans. Spanish food has European influences and is very different from the staples seen in many Central American countries.[2]

Asian cultures and their relationship to food may be summed up by a Confucian saying cited in an Ohio State University fact sheet: "A man cannot be too serious about his eating, for food is the force that binds society together."[3] Composition of meals and cooking techniques are key elements of the diverse cultures of the Asian regions. Eating involves ceremony. In Japanese culture, the appearance of food is very important.

I could list pages of different foods and cultures and explore the meanings of those foods to its people. The point is that your cultural roots affect the specific foods you eat, when you eat, and why you eat.

thing without a feast. So forget the cake-and-punch idea. It had to be an all-out meal that people would remember and talk about years later. If not, it would be an embarrassment to my family.

My parents, who had a bit more wisdom about these events than I did, reminded me that my wedding wasn't all about me, but included feeding our guests and providing them with a great meal for their participation in this momentous event. A wedding was a celebration after all. I understood and so consented to the meal. In fact, it felt rather biblical. I mean if Jesus cared enough to honor his mother's request to turn water into wine at a wedding in order to bless the guests, who was I to argue with this?

Since ancient days, regardless of religion or culture, food has been used in wedding celebrations around the world. In China, wedding food includes lobster and chicken, representing the Yin and Yang of the newly joined family. Koreans serve noodles at weddings because they symbolize longevity; in Italian weddings the shape of the bow-tied fried sugared dough treats represents good luck, and the traditional Italian wedding cake is made from biscuits, according to the

Department of Food Science at Melbourne, Australia's RMIT University.[4] And a southern African-American wedding may feature fried chicken, candied sweet potatoes, buttermilk biscuits, and seasoned mixed greens. Used at celebrations, foods can bring a common identity to groups as well. It can strengthen community and symbolize meaningful events and rituals.

The problem comes when we overindulge at those celebrations and don't listen to our bodies—*when the food becomes a fixation rather than a celebration of culture*. It's not that food and celebration are a poor pairing. What becomes problematic is our inability to enjoy the gathering without overindulging. If we become lost in the eating, we are no longer celebrating people, the event, or an important milestone.

Don't Let Celebrations Be about Your Food Struggle

One woman I know dreads going to baby showers because she always overeats at these affairs—which is easy to do. From the beginning of the event to the finish, her entire focus is on resisting the cakes and candied treats that always appear at these functions.

She is so obsessed about denying herself these treats that she can't relax and celebrate the upcoming birth with the mother-to-be. She has completely lost sight of the celebration. For her, a baby shower is all about resisting the food.

This woman needs a *press pause* moment to think about why she goes to baby showers. She is there to celebrate with the mom-to-be. When her focus changes to celebrating the mother and baby, she will be able to shift her attention to the people in the room and away from the food. Food will no longer be the centerpiece and she can better control her eating.

Because food is usually served at celebrations, she must learn to think of food and celebration as a positive thing. To do so requires rethinking why she attends baby showers. It is a celebration of a meaningful event in a friend's or relative's life.

Next, she has to stop denying herself by thinking of all the food at the celebration as "bad food." If she enjoyed a treat and stopped eating when she was satisfied, the stress of the celebration would be removed. Food becomes a part of the bigger picture. It has its place but is no longer the main event.

The message here is that food and celebration must be thought of in positive ways. We don't have to dread going to a wedding, a baby shower, a birthday party, or any other event when we keep in mind the purpose of the celebration. Food enhances these events but is not the sole reason we gather.

Alternatives to Food as a Reward

"Come on, you can do it. You can go in the potty. Hurray! You did it. Such a big boy! Here's an M&M."

"Wow, you read three books this month. Here's the free pizza coupon you earned for the reading reward!"

"All As on that report card? Time for a big ice cream sundae."

"Bob, you've worked hard all week. Let's go get a good steak dinner."

"These moms have put in so much time at the PTA meetings. I'm bringing doughnuts to our next meeting to thank them."

Every day, without people being aware of it, food and reward are tied together. No one in the above examples is intentionally trying to create problems. They just aren't thinking about the association they are creating with food as reward. And with an obesity epidemic in both kids and adults, we've got to *press pause* and think about this.

When we use food as rewards, we counter the healthy nutrition we are trying to teach our kids. It's like telling a child not to use drugs and then handing him a cigarette!

Food rewards are immediate consequences for behaviors we want to reinforce. But food also trains bad habits—eating when you aren't hungry and using food to improve behavior.

There are better ways of rewarding one another without contributing to poor health and overconsumption of unhealthy foods. You could supply lots of hugs and praise for potty training, time at a video arcade for book reading, a new basketball for good grades, a massage for the stress of hard work, a handwritten thank-you note to the moms in the PTA, and a relaxing bath before bed. All of these are as effective as food rewards. And none of them teaches us to eat when we aren't hungry or increases our preference for sweets or fatty foods!

When we think about how often we use food as a reward, we might be surprised at how routine it has become in our everyday lives. Fortunately, the habit can be broken.

Just *press pause*. Attend to the times you use food as a reward. To break the habit, jot down what makes you feel good that doesn't involve food. List ten or twenty things and hang the list on your refrigerator. The next time you want a reward, choose something from that list that doesn't involve food.

You can do the same with your kids. Instead of buying them candy or giving them treats for appropriate behavior, develop a grab bag of inexpensive items, such as stickers and small toys. Use the grab bag, not food, to reward them. Consider using activities and your time and attention as rewards, such as story time with Dad, helping Mom plant a garden, going in-line skating, having a friend spend the night, staying up fifteen minutes later, extra playtime, and so forth.

Changing rewards from food to activities such as a hot bath, a golf outing, or time with a friend will help you gradually lose the association of food and reward. It's not that you can *never* give yourself a food reward, but that you use other rewards as often as possible. Using food as a reward may interfere with reading your natural hunger cues. And our goal is to eat at scheduled meal and snack times and when hungry, not because we earned a treat.

What Happens When You Use Food as Punishment

Food is sometimes withheld as punishment. You may have been told, "Until you follow directions, no snack" or "Because you hit your sister, go to bed without dinner." Not being allowed to eat can confuse your body and mind. When this happens, it is more difficult to trust your body because you weren't allowed to eat when hungry. And if someone is deprived of treats, it makes them desire them all the more. This is at the root of all dieting struggles. You punish your body by denying it, but this approach doesn't work.

You're getting a very negative message when denied food: that you won't be fed because you are bad. Some of us are still carrying that message around in our head from childhood, and reinforcing it by our dieting mentality. *If I eat this, I'm bad,* or, *If I allow myself this treat, I don't deserve it. I'm unworthy.* Giving food the power to determine your worth is a problem. Your worth has nothing to do with food. Food is to sustain and nourish you, not punish you. So you must never believe that eating makes you "bad." Your body was designed for food.

In some cases, this message of food and punishment is so ingrained that we eat to punish ourselves. We think, *I'm not good enough to be thinner,* or, *I deserve to be fat because I am unworthy of better things.* We give up. We compare ourselves to others and feel inadequate. This has to stop! Whatever led to you feeling unworthy had nothing to do with food. You might have been teased because of your weight but your feeling of badness comes from believing the negative things people said to you. Don't allow food or weight to determine your worth. God esteems you because he created and chose you. You are loved and valued. If you can accept God's love for you, it will counter the belief that you need to be punished.

Punishment can be a self-imposed sentence learned from childhood or come from other false beliefs or traumatic experiences. So quit punishing yourself by denying your body food and falsely connecting food to your goodness or badness. If you feel condemned or inadequate, the root of this is not eating. God never intended food to be used to punish you.

Food is a provision, a blessing. The problematic pairing of food with reward or punishment can warp the meaning we give to food. Again, rethink the positive meaning of food—sustenance, nourishment, provision, celebration, connection, and community.

When Food Becomes a Control Issue

It may sound odd to talk about food as control because most of us feel out of control with food. But to many people, such as Danielle, food is all about control.

Danielle grew up in a very unpredictable home, with an alcoholic father and a frequently depressed mother. When Danielle's father was drinking, sometimes he would be quiet and calm, and other times loud and verbally abusive. Danielle's mother was equally unpredictable. Something would trigger a depressive episode and she would lock herself in her bedroom for days. Danielle felt helpless and powerless in coping with her mother's depression. She was frightened for her mother's safety and afraid to be alone with her father.

Danielle felt her life was out of control and that she was helpless to do anything about it. What she could control was her eating. When she felt anxious or upset, she binged on food in the pantry, and when overeating made her feel sick, she forced herself to vomit. This became a pattern and a source of false control in her life. As long as she could control the food by bingeing and vomiting, she could pretend to manage her life. The problem came when the bingeing and vomiting began to control her. Tired and worried about the toll her eating behavior was having on her body, she contacted a therapist in order to learn how to stop using food in this controlling way.

In the beginning, food was Danielle's way of controlling her unpredictable world. Now food was controlling her and it lost all real meaning of nourishment and sustenance. Food became her enemy and the source of her struggles.

Danielle, like so many other people, began to use food in the wrong manner because she saw it as a means of control in an uncontrolled family. Until she developed an awareness of the meaning she had given to food, change was not coming. She had unintentionally linked food to control, and it eventually controlled her. Healing began when she assigned food its proper value—a source of nourishment to be enjoyed and used to sustain her.

Erin, on the other hand, was envious of her beautiful teenaged daughter, who was often complimented for her beauty. While Erin felt proud of her daughter, she also felt envious of her youthful body. Erin, at midlife, could not compete with her daughter's cellulite-free legs, firm arms, flat stomach, and toned upper body. Even though Erin ate well and exercised, midlife changes a woman's body. This is simply part of the aging process Erin was unwilling to accept.

Plus, Erin's marriage was on shaky ground, younger women were rising in the ranks at work, and her career goals were yet to be fulfilled. Control and identity were at the center of her body dissatisfaction.

In order to cope with life changes and aging, Erin developed an unhealthy relationship with food. Feeling out of control in so many areas of her life, Erin was determined to get her shape back to that of a twenty-year-old. She began to control every bite of food that went into her mouth. She denied physical cues of hunger and did sit-ups after she ate. Food became her enemy—the thing that stood between her and her fantasy of turning back the clock. Eventually, Erin developed anorexia.

Erin's struggle with food had everything to do with accepting that which she could not control and knowing where her true identity was found. Food had nothing to do with either. Food was the vehicle used to act out feelings of control and insecurity. Once Erin realized that her identity was not tied to accomplishments and outward beauty, she began to explore her identity in God with the help of a therapist. Already accepted and unconditionally loved, God didn't care if her physical body aged. He was concerned about her heart. And he, along with a therapist, was willing to listen to her fears and anxieties.

Relinquishing control over those things we can't control is necessary in all our lives. We will be held accountable for our *reactions* to uncontrollable events, not whether or not we could prevent them from happening. To develop a healthy relationship with food, Erin had to surrender the food and tackle the tough issues in her life. Food was not her enemy.

Make Your Relationship with Food a Positive One

It is up to you to think about the meaning of food in your life. The meaning you give food often determines how you use it. Once you've identified that meaning, you can keep it or change it. A healthy way to think about food is that it is something enjoyable, not cursed. Food brings life. It is to be experienced, not avoided or rushed through to make life easier. Food serves a needed purpose and satisfies our physical hunger. It connects us to our cultural identity and is part of celebration.

The Italian proverb *La vita e incerta mangia il dolce per primo* means "Life is uncertain, eat dessert first." Why wait for the main course when you can enjoy it all! The point is we can enjoy eating and still be healthy.

I find the Italian exuberance for life infectious, whether it's having an intimate dinner with family or friends, laughing, joking, or just being together. Friends of mine have a small house in a tiny rural village near Tuscany, and every holiday they enter a world in which eating is celebrated, not considered an act of guilt and anxiety. Quite refreshing! When it comes to eating, we all need a taste of this in our lives. We don't want to become one of the growing number of people who eat more but enjoy food less. Instead, let's honor the gift of food and our bodies and develop a peaceful eating relationship with food.

THE PRESS PAUSE PRINCIPLE

Purpose to reflect on the meaning you give to eating and food.

Attend to any negative meanings you give food, such as reward, punishment, control.

Understand the role culture, family, and recent history play in the way you view eating and food right now.

Strategize ways to change your negative views of food and eating (don't pair it with reward, don't use it to punish yourself, and don't use it to control things that feel out of control).

Execute changes:
  ▷ Embrace eating as celebration, connection, and a reflection of culture identity.
  ▷ Substitute other behaviors as rewards for appropriate behaviors and healthy functioning.
  ▷ Surrender control. You don't have it anyway. You have control only over your reactions to events, people, and things.

PAUSE FOR WISDOM
Nothing would be more tiresome than eating and drinking if God had not made them a pleasure as well as a necessity.
VOLTAIRE

6

RELAX AND PUT DOWN THE FORK

Have you ever munched your way through a bag of chips or dug into the ice cream and looked down and realized you'd eaten nearly the whole container? Perhaps you race through a meal without tasting a bite because you feel tense and worried about a problem at work or a family issue.

If so, consider yourself in good company. You are doing what so many of us do—stress eat. Food calms us down. We don't mean to use food this way but we do. It is almost an unconscious act. Stressed—we eat. Tense—we eat.

I attended a women's retreat at a beach house on the oceanfront, and each woman was asked to bring a snack to share. Because I am an eating disorder therapist, I decided to bring something healthy. I brought fruit.

Let me tell you, I was alone in my thinking. The amount of chocolate that showed up at this retreat was enough to feed the beach community and throw a party for the city! As each woman arrived, pounds of chocolate were laid on the beach house tables. It was decadent, delectable, and strangely . . . relaxing. Yes, relaxing. Just knowing the chocolate was available and ready for immediate consumption de-stressed most of us. Clearly, chocolate was our weekend friend!

As I scanned the chocolate-laden table stockpiled with many of my favorite treats, I flashed back to when I was a child living near the shores of Lake Michigan. I remembered the hot summer days when the ice cream truck sang its way through my neighborhood. Parents found the truck annoying but to kids, it was heaven.

We'd rush to the open window of the big yellow truck, ready to sample one of those pictured treats we'd all memorized from the posters plastered on the sides—Fudgsicles, Push-Ups, Creamsicles, Drumsticks, and other treats. Those treats and the carefree days of summer were a delightful pairing. And that pairing has followed me into adult life. Many of us have these same associations. We pair certain foods with stress reduction. So when we need a carefree moment, we pull out the comfort food that reminds us of pleasant memories or takes us away for a moment.

A survey by the American Psychological Association found that one in four people in the United States turns to food for comfort when they feel down or stressed. During holidays, that number jumps to one in three people.[1] To stop mindless eating, we need to understand the connection between stress and eating.

Why We Want Certain Foods

Men and women both reach for ice cream in times of stress, but otherwise their comfort food choices diverge. Women eat more in response to stress than men, and tend to crave sweets. (Did we really need research to tell us this?) Men prefer hot dishes such as pizza, casseroles, and steak when tension rises.[2]

A University of California–Davis study suggests that this difference is because of personality traits and early childhood associations. One theory is that men like heartier comfort foods because these

Why We All Reach for Ice Cream

When men and women were polled in a *Psychology Today* study, their number one comfort food was ice cream.[3] And pleasant memories of days gone by aren't the only reason we reach for this treat. Foods high in fat and sugar physically calm us when we feel lonely or stressed. This isn't our imagination: Research at the University of California–San Francisco indicates that these confections relieve negative emotions better than other foods. These studies suggest that high-energy sugary foods eaten during chronic stress tell the brain to calm down.[4] And when we need our brains to calm down, ice cream is our first choice.

So all those movies you've watched in which you see the characters go to the freezer, pull out the pints of ice cream, and eat their way through a broken romance or a horrible day are right on target.

The trick for you is to *press pause* and try an alternative such as a walk around the block, a hot bath, or a healthy snack before digging into the ice cream.

But if ice cream is the only thing that will suffice, put one or two scoops in an attractive small bowl or sherbet dish—and enjoy every bite.

foods remind them of their mothers' cooking (mashed potatoes, meat, soups, and so forth). Because women associate these foods with too much work, we go for the easy fixes like chocolate and sweets. A study at the University of Illinois suggests that we reach for different comfort foods at different times, depending on our mood.

My father likes meat-and-potatoes meals. I have a good relationship with my father and many happy memories. So when I cook meals with meat and potatoes, it reminds me of sitting around the dinner table as a child enjoying family time—a pleasant experience. Food was a big part of that pleasant experience.

My husband likes meat and potatoes and the way I fix them. He feels nurtured with this type of meal and associates it with me taking care of him. As an adult, he is comforted by my hearty meals.

My mom baked pies with fresh berries—incredible pies! They were a labor of love that she presented to her family. So pies comfort me. They remind me of Mom's love and care for me.

Even though both men and women use comfort foods to de-stress, we choose different foods and respond differently to the experience. According to another University of Illinois study,[5] men choose protein-dense foods to increase positive emotions. Women prefer high-calorie sweet snacks such as chocolate and ice cream when feeling down and stressed. The problem is that after consuming these mood enhancers, according to a Cornell study, women feel guilty, not happy like the men.[6]

But comforting yourself this way only works momentarily. After indulging, you engage in painful self-judgment: *How could you be so weak?* Stress hormones kick back up and you crave the comfort food again. You eat and feel better until the guilt of what you have done sets in. It's a vicious cycle.

To stop this cycle, *press pause* and become aware of what you are doing. Instead of using comfort foods, take steps to fix the source of the stress or to de-stress in more positive ways. To calm down, you might get a quick neck rub, take a short walk, or sit quietly in a room. To attack the source of the stress, take action. For example, if you are in debt, enroll in a budgeting class; if you are upset with a relative, decide to confront that person; if you feel ignored in your marriage, go to marriage counseling. More ideas are presented throughout this chapter.

Sources of Stress

If we categorized stress, we could pinpoint it as coming from three areas: events that happen; things we do to ourselves, and our relationships (this one is covered in chapter 14).

Events that happen. We feel frustration when something gets in the way of our goals. We can't find a job that pays enough to buy a house; the movie we wanted to see is sold out; the dry cleaners lost the outfit we needed for a wedding; we are late and have a flat tire. These and similar experiences can result in stress, and if we don't know how to deal with these interruptions and frustrations, we may eat to calm ourselves.

Lynne was driving to work when there was a detour on her usual route. All she could think about was how late she was going to be. Her heart started pounding and she could feel herself growing tense with every slowdown of traffic. She began munching on a bag of chips. By the time she reached the end of the detour, she had eaten the entire bag.

Things don't always go the way we want them to go. Problems are a fact of life. Instead of stressing out over what we can't change (such as a detour), we can shift our focus to what we can control—our expectations and reactions.

It's not realistic to expect our day to go smoothly, with no bumps in the road. Life throws us curves and takes twists and turns. Our ability to be flexible, to be confident that we can cope when inevitable frustrations come, is vital to reducing stress.

God didn't promise us a life without frustrations or difficulties. Instead he promises to be with us through difficulty, to give us a peace that we can't fully explain. If we believe the promises of God, we can trust God for the outcome of any frustrating situation and remain faithful in our response because we know that he is with us.

From a spiritual perspective, difficulty can be used for our own good. It matures us, sharpens us, and brings a new compassion for others. Maybe a detour in the road put us in touch with a person in need. Maybe a delay was divine and prevented us from disaster. When we think about delays and interruptions in a positive way, we don't feel tense or stressed.

On a flight home from Atlanta, I was looking forward to quietly reading. I opened my book but it soon became evident that the elderly man next to me wanted to talk. I gave him numerous nonverbal signals that I didn't want to talk, but finally gave in and listened to him. Alone, struggling with a chronic illness, he felt hopeless.

The lady in the seat in front of us asked if she could join the conversation. It turned out she was having similar symptoms. She was very thankful to have people to talk to about these issues. We ended the flight with hope.

Initially I had been annoyed with the intrusion into my quiet time. But the intrusion was purposeful. Two people on that flight needed advice and encouragement. There was purpose in the interruption and I was able to help people in need.

What we do to ourselves. Some stress is self-imposed, when we feel pressure to meet the unrealistic expectations of others or when we put unrealistic expectations on ourselves. No one can live up to standards of perfection. People with eating disorders often don't give themselves permission to make mistakes or fail. They don't see their strengths and instead focus on perceived weaknesses. Overall, their expectations are so high they can't meet them and feel inadequate. Feelings of inadequacy or low self-worth lead to overeating.

Carrie wanted desperately to do well in school and felt she could distinguish herself if she was at the top of her class. She became extremely competitive with others and mentally berated herself if she received a B on any homework assignment. She spent hours studying and gave up any hope for a social life. She defined herself by success. Any mistake meant she was "bad" or inadequate.

Like many people, Carrie began to use food to calm herself down. To deal with tension, she ate. When she started gaining weight, she decided to vomit in order to rid herself of the food.

Carrie never intended to develop bulimia but that is what she did. At the root of her problem were unrealistic expectations related to self-imposed stress. Carrie needed help defining herself apart from accomplishments and performance. Part of that process was to embrace realistic expectations for herself and to learn that her true identity was not found in what she accomplished.

Coping with Metabolic Stress

Let's say that work has been especially difficult. You've got a deadline and time is running out. You grab a caramel macchiato and a candy bar to keep up your energy during the day. You have to get this project done. But what is happening to your body after you down all that caffeine and sugar to make the deadline?

Your blood sugar spikes. Your pancreas secretes a lot of insulin to normalize your blood sugar. Then your blood sugar level drops and you feel tired and lethargic. The low blood sugar level makes you feel hungry and you crave sugar and gulp down another sugar-loaded coffee.

The average person consumes thirty-one teaspoons of sugar a day—nineteen more than the recommended *maximum* of twelve teaspoons established by the U.S. Department of Agriculture's Food Guide Pyramid. Most of us are loading our bodies with too much sugar. Our bodies are stressed just from the amount of sugar that our blood glucose levels have to contend with on a regular basis. Noticed I said the *amount* of sugar. This is important because studies show that when under stress a little sugar calms you down and won't lead to that dreaded weight gain.

The concern about eating large amounts of refined sugar is that the rapid fluctuations of blood sugar levels stress the body. So the next time you feel the pressure of that deadline, reach for a whole-grain cracker with cheese or peanut butter instead of a soda (which has about eight to ten teaspoons of sugar).

You don't have to cut out all sugar in your diet—just cut back. Sugar is in many foods you wouldn't expect, such as ketchup, so read labels on processed foods and adjust your intake. Eliminating or cutting back on sodas will make a difference. You will also want to avoid high-fructose corn syrup in particular, which has been linked to weight gain. Watch your portions and try to satisfy that sweet craving with fruit or a small amount of dessert.

When you need an energy boost, *press pause* and reach for a healthy snack—one that won't play havoc with your blood sugar levels, such as fresh vegetables, whole grains, cheese, or other protein. And watch your intake of caffeine.

According to Duke University Medical Center researchers, caffeine can enhance your stress levels, so moderate your caffeine levels when you are under stress.[7] Other research is mixed on the pros and cons of caffeine, but caffeine does increase blood pressure, heart rate, and stress hormone levels.

Think about how unhealthy food stresses your body metabolically. Good nutrition can help remove or reduce that stress. Consider healthful ways of reenergizing, such as getting up from your desk and taking a brisk walk, perhaps up and down stairs. Make smart choices with snacks and energy boosts during your day to avoid stressing the body more than necessary. Plan ahead so you have healthy snacks on hand.

Getting enough sleep is a part of de-stressing the body as well. Ever had someone tell you, "Don't lose sleep over it"? It's good advice.

Studies show that when we don't get enough sleep, hormonal changes contribute to increased risk for high blood pressure and diabetes.[8] We need that eight hours of sleep experts recommend to keep our stress levels down, according to researchers from the University of Chicago Medical Center.

The Body and Brain Partnership

Let's look specifically at what is happening in our bodies under stress. According to Georgetown University Medical Center's stress expert Mary Dallman, PhD, when we feel stressed by something or someone, our bodies naturally kick into gear.[9] The hormone cortisol elevates and tells our bodies to get ready to handle stress. Our hearts begin to race, we become alert, blood vessels constrict, and muscles prepare to act. Once the stress passes, cortisol also tells the brain to stop producing it.

But when we are under chronic stress, our brain just keeps producing more cortisol, often causing anxiety and depression. During all of this, other parts of the brain tell us to start looking for high-energy foods, which are high in fat and sugar to help us survive the stress.

The cortisol directs the fat from these extra calories to our abdomens so it can be used effectively for energy. Then those fat stores tell the brain to stop the process and turn off the cortisol.

Researcher Sarah Leibowitz at Rockefeller University found that the urge to stress-eat may be related to the timing of the stress. If we eat carbs with no muscular activity to use those carbs, says a *Psychology Today* article reporting her work, stress sends the carbs directly to fat storage.[10]

But we aren't doomed to reach for the comfort food every time we feel stressed! Exercise, prayer and meditation, soothing music, and hot baths help keep stress at bay and shut off the chronic stress mechanism by stimulating the same pleasure centers in the brain—without using food.

How Stressful Thoughts Hurt Us

Our thoughts are very important when it comes to managing stress-eating. Thoughts influence feelings, which influence the way we act.

Our actions influence our perceptions. Our perceptions influence our thoughts, and the cycle repeats.

Getting control of our thoughts is essential to better living. An important truth is that stress is not intolerable. No matter how bad a situation looks, with God's help, you can handle it. This is his promise to us. He won't give us more than we can handle. I know this sounds like a nice cliché and please don't quote it to people in the middle of difficulty. No one who is deeply troubled likes to hear clichés. Better to help the person focus his or her thoughts on the One who can help us through difficult times. If we do this, we can learn to tolerate stress without crunching our way through toffee buttered popcorn.

Let me give you an example from my own life. For seven years my husband and I had no discernible reason why we couldn't have children. We were part of the small percentage of couples whose infertility was undefined. Not only were we not getting pregnant, but no doctor could tell us why it hadn't happening.

I had no reason to think I wouldn't easily become pregnant. And because doctors insisted it could happen, I made up all kinds of reasons in my head why it hadn't. Some of these reasons were reinforced by friends who had no idea what they were talking about. I was told that my infertility was a punishment from God for past sins, that sin in my life was keeping me from getting pregnant, that there was a generational curse on me, and that I lacked faith in God. None of these things were true, but when you are stressed, you may believe almost anything you wouldn't normally consider. Stress makes you vulnerable to stinking thinking.

The longer the infertility lasted, the more negative my thoughts were. I believed I was inadequate, a failure, and couldn't do what most women take for granted. The battle I fought was in my mind. And the negative thoughts along with the misguided voices of others left me stressed and depressed.

I had trouble sleeping, felt like crying for no reason, became irritable, and wanted to isolate myself. I couldn't bear seeing women pregnant at the mall, had difficulty attending friends' baby showers, and felt like my life was out of control.

Every month, I would hope and pray for conception and then be gravely disappointed. Then I did conceive but miscarried. Over a seven-year period, this stress became almost unbearable. Had I not been an eating disorder therapist, I would have eaten my way through this time. I watched a number of my infertile friends turn to food for comfort. Instead I chose to take care of my body and not increase stress on it by overeating or eating poorly. It wasn't an easy choice, more like a daily surrender.

More important, I had to align my thoughts with what I knew to be true based on my faith. God wasn't punishing me for past sins. I wasn't living a willfully sinful life, nor was I under a curse. And because there was no medical reason for my infertility, I had immense faith that God could open my womb and I could conceive.

As I examined my thoughts and challenged my beliefs, I concluded that my stress and anxiety were based on faulty thinking. I had to refocus on what I considered to be my core beliefs. God is trustworthy and had my best interest in mind. My response was to surrender to his will and trust his faithfulness.

I can now look back on that time and understand the maturity and growth God brought through those seven years. I learned surrender, compassion for others, and to trust what I cannot see—the basis of faith. In his time, God brought me children. And my appreciation for them is tremendous because of the anguish I experienced before their arrival. God knew what he was doing all along. When my thoughts and heart lined up with what I knew to be true—that God loved me and cared about my plight—my stress diminished.

We live in a world in which bad things happen. I don't always understand why things happen the way they do, but I have learned to trust God. When I revisited my core beliefs at that time of infertility, a sense of peace enveloped me and the need to eat diminished. I still had to grieve my loss and I still have unanswered questions, but the source of my stress was gone. When the source of stress is removed, stress-eating is no longer needed.

Reducing and Preventing Stress

There are times when stress can be reduced or even prevented. The more you can do either, the less likely you will stress-eat.

John liked to spend money on things he couldn't afford. When the bills piled up, John began to relieve his stress through nightly snacking. He felt like he couldn't stop eating.

At a friend's suggestion, John saw a financial counselor to establish a budget and pay off creditors; he made an appointment with a mental health counselor as well. He realized his need to buy material things was driven by feelings of inadequacy. If he didn't address his thoughts of not being good enough, he would go back to food for comfort. Spending was only a symptom of a deeper belief he held about himself.

The financial counselor sorted through his money mess and made plans for debt relief. The mental health counselor addressed his thoughts of inadequacy. John eventually stopped stress-eating. In this case, the source of John's stress was removed.

Many of us could benefit from asking, *Is it possible to reduce any of the stress in my life? Could I cut out an activity, learn to solve problems better, get enough sleep, say no to more responsibility, exercise more, or learn to be more assertive?*

Of course you can't reduce or eliminate all stress from your life. You can't tell cancer to go away or an irritating mother-in-law to leave you alone for the rest of your life. I couldn't stop being infertile for seven years. Certain stresses will be with us, and we must learn to cope with them without using food to calm down. So let's do this: Let's agree that stress can be tolerated. This may take a little faith but try to embrace this idea. Each time you feel stress in the day, acknowledge the stressful event or trigger and notice your urge to eat. I do this when I write.

When I write a book, I sit at a computer for hours during the day. To me, this is stressful. I like to be up and active, not tied to a screen. I often find myself reaching for food even though I am not hungry.

I used to keep a bowl of M&Ms at my desk. Not smart. I love M&Ms and don't just eat a few when they are sitting in front of me. I switched to grapes but then realized that grapes—which have many health benefits, but are quite high in natural sugar—weren't doing the trick. I needed calming food or no food at all. The best choice was no food.

I also needed a new strategy. So I decided to redirect my thoughts: *I feel stressed sitting at this desk all day. I can tolerate this. It's a part of writing a book Instead of eating, I need to get up and walk around the room or take a break outside. During my lunch hour, I can make a trip to the gym and work out. The last thing I need to do is sit and inhale candy. The crunch of the M&Ms is satisfying. The sugar and fat calm me down temporarily, but then I feel bad and gain weight. Noshing and nibbling are not good stress reducers for me. I also need to remove the M&Ms from my desk!*

Let's break this down. First, I acknowledged the stress: I don't like to sit for hours on end doing something that takes great concentration. This is true. But I need to add to my thoughts and say, *I'm a grown-up and this is my job, so I need to do this. I can do this.*

Second, food is only *one* way to relieve tension. I need to find other ways to reduce my stress. Exercise works for me. Lose the M&Ms and go for a brief walk.

The point is, I had to change my thoughts from, *Oh, no, I'm doomed because I have to sit for days on end in front of a computer and that is stressful,* to *I can do this if I plan healthy ways to reduce my stress.* Positive thoughts lead to positive action. Our thoughts are not only important in managing stress, but in many other areas that involve eating. Because of this, I've devoted all of chapter 10 to the power of thoughts.

Other ways to reduce stress include learning and practicing simple relaxation techniques. Deep breathing and deep muscle relaxation are two easy ones to add to your de-stressing toolbox.

Deep breathing. When you concentrate on taking deep, slow breaths, you supply more oxygen to the brain and muscle system. You stimulate the parasympathetic nervous system, which calms you. Taking deep breaths can help you clear your mind.

When you are tense, breathing often becomes short and rapid. It tends to originate in the chest. Some people even hyperventilate, which can lead to panic. Breathing should come from the abdomen, not the chest. If you are unsure where you are breathing from, place your hand on your abdomen, take a breath, and see if your hand moves. If you don't feel an in-and-out motion, chances are you are breathing from your chest and throat.

To practice deep breathing, concentrate on your body. Inhale slowly through your nose and let the air go down low. Pause and slowly exhale through your nose.

Using this technique, breathe in and out about ten times. When you practice deep breathing three or four times a day, you will catch yourself breathing incorrectly and teach your body to breathe correctly. The good thing about this form of relaxation is that it is free, easy, and can be done anywhere. If you are in the middle of a crowd and start feeling tense, you can take a number of deep, slow breaths to calm down. Or you can practice alone in your home. Or do both!

Deep muscle relaxation. If you tend to carry stress in your body or are prone to tension in your head, neck, shoulders, or back, try deep muscle relaxation, which is based on the idea that tensing a muscle and then releasing it produces a state of relaxation.

First, find a comfortable and quiet place to practice. Start with a muscle and tense it. Wait a few seconds (study the tension), release the muscle, and feel the relaxation (for about fifteen seconds). Repeat this with all muscle groups, including your stomach, head (eyes, mouth, jaw), triceps, back, legs, feet, and biceps. Make sure no tension creeps in when you practice. Concentrate on each muscle and clear your head of other thoughts.

You should practice for about twenty minutes per day. It usually takes about twenty to thirty minutes to go through all the muscle groups and become completely relaxed. Good times to practice are when the alarm goes off in the morning and right before bed at night. This way, you start your day calm and end it the same way. Practicing at night also helps you fall asleep.

Lessons from the Couch

All the years I was in clinical practice I had a couch in my therapy room. Despite the stereotype of having patients lie down on the couch, they rarely used it. But when someone requested treatment for stress-related issues, I wanted to see how well they could relax their physical body. So I would often ask clients to lie down on my couch, get as comfortable as possible, and relax their bodies as best they could. Then I would ask the person to rate his or her relaxation level on a scale from 1 to 10—one being so tense they could hardly breathe, and ten being so relaxed they felt almost medicated.

Typically, a stressed person appeared physically tense: tightened face, pursed lips, tense arms and legs, and so forth. But this person would give a rating of 8 or above on my 10-point scale.

This person believed he was very relaxed. However, the person's body was saying the opposite. He had no awareness of how much tension was physically carried in the body. To me, he looked more like a 2 or 3 on that 10-point scale. The physical signs of tension were easy to read.

What I realized from this exercise was that tension was a natural state for many people. They simply were not aware of how much tension they carried in their bodies day to day. A state of body relaxation was foreign. Tension and stress were their normal states.

Why? These clients had a common history. Most of them were raised in families with chaos, unpredictability, and little or no structure, some with a parent or both parents alcoholic, abusive, mentally ill, or disorganized. These clients never knew what to expect from day to day or even hour to hour. This unpredictability and lack of structure left them feeling anxious and uptight most of the time.

Relaxation was foreign because they spent their childhoods never knowing what to expect next. This created daily tension and worry. Would Dad come home drunk? Would Mom be depressed and unresponsive? Would Dad be verbally abusive? Would Mom scream for no apparent reason? Would the house be a mess? Would we have dinner? These stressful thoughts and experiences resulted in body tension. The more unpredictable the home, the more tension the person seemed to carry.

Even those of us who haven't been to therapy can relate to living our lives in a chronic state of tension. If you watch the news, listen to the radio, or scan the Internet, you are aware that stress is a part of modern-day life. Our rushed, tense, unpredictable, and disorganized lives combined with uncertainty in the world can result in a chronic state of tension. We worry about safety, school shootings, terrorist attacks, our bills, hurricanes, tornados, our marriage, the choices our children make, our elderly parents, health care, illnesses . . . the list is long. And this tension affects our eating.

Learning to De-Stress

We must learn to recognize the signs of stress because stress registers on the body, usually before the mind tunes in to it. Both body and mind are working together, but we may not notice it. To avoid mindless eating, we need to be conscious of the stress in our bodies.

So how do we calm down without using food as our agent? It might be useful to keep a stress diary to help you connect stressful events to physical symptoms. This is nothing more than a written record of a stressful event or cue and how you responded to it. For example, if your boss is an upsetting person and calls you into her office only when there is a problem, make a note of your physical reaction the next time you get called in to see her. Did you have a slight headache or a tightness in your stomach?

If you experience one or more of the following symptoms after an event or trigger, you could be experiencing signs of stress.

- ▶ Aching back
- ▶ Headaches
- ▶ Nervous stomach
- ▶ Tense shoulders
- ▶ Clenched hands
- ▶ Rapid heartbeat
- ▶ Shortness of breath
- ▶ Difficulty falling asleep
- ▶ Sleeping too much
- ▶ Muscle tension
- ▶ Cold hands and feet
- ▶ Diarrhea or constipation
- ▶ Ulcers
- ▶ Grinding teeth
- ▶ Skin problems
- ▶ Appetite changes
- ▶ Overeating

You should check with a physician to see if these are stress related rather than some other condition.

Stress also can present symptoms such as depression, anxiety, poor concentration, forgetfulness, feeling overwhelmed or driven, mood swings, crying spells, irritability, agitation, obsessing, compulsive behavior, guilt, worry, temper problems, sexual difficulty, nightmares, boredom, and apathy. Because stress can lead to physical and psychological symptoms, it needs to be reduced or managed. And we don't want to keep using food to cope. It's better to rethink the way we react to life.

So before I discuss ways to help you tolerate stress, based on everything we've read so far, take this brief stress test and see how you score. The questions to which you answer yes indicate stress in your life, which may affect your eating.

1. When you are tense or uptight, do you crave sugar or salty foods?
2. When you feel a lack of energy or are tired, do you reach for caffeine or sugar to keep yourself going?
3. Do you feel tension and stress but don't know how to relieve those feelings?
4. Do you eat fast food because you are too busy to stop and make a meal?
5. Do you feel exhausted at the end of the day but feel you are too busy to exercise?
6. Do you find yourself skipping meals because you are too busy?
7. Are you gaining weight but feel your eating plan hasn't really changed?
8. Do you sleep less than seven hours a night?
9. Do you notice more weight around your middle?
10. Do you eat when you are not hungry but feel nervous or tense?

How to Combat Stress-Eating

The goal is to stop being overwhelmed by stress and to learn positive strategies (nonfood) to deal with it. If you are a stress-eater, try these options:

Delay eating for twenty minutes. Most cravings will pass if you can distract yourself from the food.

Write down what you eat in a day. Keep that stress diary we discussed. Any time you keep track of what you put in your mouth, you become more aware and mindful of eating. This usually results in eating less.

Change your routine. I exercise midday because that is the time of day I feel the most stressed from sitting all morning. I used to go to the gym early morning (to get it over with) but realized I need the break (and those increased endorphins) midday.

Eat at the table and don't do anything else. When you are stressed, it's easy to mindlessly eat when doing something else because you are "saving time." Usually this means you'll eat more or eat unconsciously.

Eat regularly. Eat at mealtimes and incorporate regular snacks during your day so you don't eat when stressed.

Pay attention to the physical sensation of hunger. If you don't feel it, pause and rethink your urge to eat.

Change your routine. If you like to reach for a venti caramel macchiato to calm you down, don't stop at that favorite coffee stand.

Remove temptation. Don't buy whatever foods seem irresistible, or remove them from sight. For instance, I can't have M&Ms sitting in a bowl when I work. I'll keep eating them if I do. They need to be out of sight or given away.

Indulge a little. If all you can think about is that square of dark chocolate when stressed, eat it. Notice I said, "Eat the square," not an entire package of squares. A little bit can satisfy the stress craving.

Evaluate the ways you de-stress. If food is your only option, you need to expand your repertoire of relaxation. Keep reading. There is more to come.

THE PRESS PAUSE PRINCIPLE

Purpose to not use food for stress relief.

Attend to your body and look for signs of tension.

Understand that chronic stress takes a toll on the body and that sugar and caffeine can stress the body metabolically.

Strategize ways to reduce, prevent, or tolerate stress better. Keep a stress diary.

Execute change by fixing the source of your stress and expanding your repertoire of relaxation.

    ▷ Take a hot bath.
    ▷ Take a walk, read a book.
    ▷ Put on soothing music.
    ▷ Pray and meditate on scripture.
    ▷ Call a friend.
    ▷ Have some hot herbal tea.

PAUSE FOR WISDOM

*Pay mind to your own life, your own health,
and wholeness. A bleeding heart is of no help
to anyone if it bleeds to death.*

FREDERICK BUECHNER

7

LOOK AROUND:
HIDDEN CUES THAT MAKE US EAT

Dinner was over and I was doing what many moms do at the end of the meal—cleaning up the dishes as kids rushed off to do homework and my husband took out the dog. As I put the leftovers in plastic containers, I noticed that there was only about a half of cup of rice left. It was too little to save and too much to throw out, so I ate it. I wasn't a bit hungry, having been satisfied by the meal I had prepared, but I ate it anyway. Why? Because it was there.

Another time I was out to dinner with friends. As we chatted, the waiter brought munchies to our table while we decided what to order. I began picking at the snacks. By the time I ordered, I had eaten a lot of snacks. Why? They were on the table and I was engaged in good conversation with great friends. I wasn't paying attention to what I was eating.

What happened to me happens to all of us every day. We eat without being aware of why. But if we think about it, a big reason we eat is because food is in front of us. The sight of it cues us to eat.

Think about the number of times you eat for this reason—the bread basket at the restaurant is on the table before the entrées are served, chips and salsa are immediately brought to the table in most Mexican restaurants, doughnuts sit by the coffeepot at the office, someone brings in fresh baked goods to the meeting, and so on.

We eat not because we are hungry, but because food is available. We "eat with our eyes," according to Brian Wansink, PhD, a food marketing psychologist at Cornell University and the executive director of the USDA's Center for Nutrition Policy and Promotion. Small things out of our awareness lure us into eating without thinking. We trust our eyes more than our stomachs. And two consequences of unintentional eating often result: We eat too much, and we eat when we aren't hungry.

If you begin to attend to these cues, you can make decisions based on a greater awareness. Small changes in your environment can help you eat with intention.

Beware of "Snack Traps"

Julie is stumped as to why she can't lose the extra twenty pounds she carries from her last pregnancy. The problem is that Julie forgets some of the things she eats, like the cookies her friend gave her at the mall, the latte she had midafternoon, the extra helping of pasta at dinner, and the late-night brownie and ice cream.

When I ask an overweight patient to give me an accounting of food eaten in a day, I ask questions such as these:

Did you taste the pasta sauce as you were cooking?
Do you pop a few pieces of candy in your mouth when you pass the candy dish in your home during the day?
Did you check the portion size on that bag of chips to see if you were eating one serving or two?

Was that a four-ounce piece of chicken on your plate or an eight-ounce piece?

When you cleaned up the dishes and pots and pans, did you eat anything?

Most people, like Julie, are unaware of the extra calories that go in their mouths without thinking. And those extra calories make a difference. A few hundred extra calories a day can prevent you from losing weight. So attend to all the times you pop a little something in your mouth.

Every day, we are cued to eat or overeat something that is out of our awareness. Our environment triggers us to eat when we are not hungry. We need to become aware of cues, to *press pause* for a moment and increase our awareness of unintentionally eating, and do what we can to make changes.

In a Cornell study conducted by Brian Wansink, PhD, and Jeffrey Sobal, PhD, participants were asked how many food decisions they made in a day. People estimated they made fourteen decisions per day. When the participants tracked their food decisions, it turned out that the average number was over *two hundred* a day.[1] That is a lot of decisions involving food! And most of those decisions are not made consciously or related to hunger, but are prompted by things in our environment.

So what external cues influence our eating decisions? We've already discussed one—that the presence and convenience of food is enough to make most of us grab that candy bar or eat that extra piece of pizza. Hunger is not our motivator. Seeing food is sometimes all it takes.

In a previous chapter, I mentioned that the smell of a food can prompt us to eat or even turn us off from eating. Temperature also influences "appetite." In this chapter, we will take a look at other common environmental cues that trigger us to eat.

Consider Ambience

Sushi is one of my favorite foods. Where I live, there are several places to enjoy this wonderful cuisine. My favorite place is an intimate spot with low lights and candles. Soft, soothing music plays quietly in the background. The room feels warm and inviting— muted earth-tone walls complement the crisp white tablecloths set with beautiful Japanese dinnerware. Waiters smile and people seem relaxed, unhurried, and engaged with their dinner partners. Enjoying sushi at this restaurant is an experience, not just a meal.

Or how about the experience you have when you walk into a Starbucks anywhere in the country? Starbucks conveys that same "pause, rest, relax, and enjoy" ambience. In fact, in 1995 a project team was formed to make Starbucks a comforting place with a sense of community.[2] Starbucks knows how to create an atmosphere that invites you to linger and have an experience. The atmosphere encourages the consumption of coffee and snacks, not to mention the cleverly packaged gifts.

Music can also influence our eating behavior. When the music is soft, we tend to eat more slowly and consume less, according to a study in *Psychology and Marketing*.[3] In restaurants with loud, disturbing music, you just want to eat and get out of there! But you tend to eat quickly and consequently too much; speedy tunes apparently make you eat faster and eat more.

So choose quiet restaurants, and when at home try eating to a relaxing CD; pay attention to how much you are actually eating. Being aware that music influences how we eat can help us moderate our eating.

Visual and situational cues encourage us to eat less or more. This doesn't mean to avoid inviting surroundings—in fact, you may eat less and enjoy your food more in a pleasant, quiet, relaxing setting. Just be aware of your surroundings.

Choose Your Plates and Glasses Carefully

When my daughter was in the musical production of *Beauty and the Beast*, she played a dancing fork. As the table settings came to life for the song "Be Our Guest," there she was in a gold unitard dancing as a large fork surrounded by dancing spoons, knives, napkins, and dinner plates.

The show was dazzling, but these larger-than-life utensils and plates reminded me that size matters when it comes to dinnerware. The bigger the dinnerware, the greater the chances we will overeat, according to an article in the *Annual Review of Nutrition*.[4] When it comes to setting our tables, bigger is not better.

Take a look at your everyday drinking glasses. You will drink less if they are tall and thin versus wide and short, according to an article in the *Journal of Consumer Research*. Studies confirm that we are tricked in our minds by the shape and size of drinking glasses.[5] Pour your drink into a tall slender glass and you'll pour less than if you pour it into a wide short glass!

According to an article in *Better Health & Living*, Lisa Young, RD, PhD, recommends using a ten-ounce glass for calorie-filled beverages rather than a twenty-ounce one.[6] The bigger the glass, the more likely we are to drink too much. The same is true of containers and packages. The bigger they are, the more we overeat, according to an article in the *Annual Review of Nutrition*. So use your short fat tumblers that hold more ounces for water, and tall slender glasses for beverages with calories.

Now, take a look at your dishes. Are they large, almost platter size? Big mistake! The bigger the dishes, the more we eat. A small portion gets lost on a big plate and looks like you have not served yourself enough food. Conversely, a nine- to ten-inch-diameter dinner plate will keep your portion size smaller than if you use a twelve-inch plate. That same serving size on a small plate looks big. Again, you might be thinking, that won't trick me. Research says differently. We are influenced by these external cues.

Consider replacing a soup spoon with a teaspoon. If you down-size, you will eat less. And the next time you grab a snack, place it in the smallest dish you have.

It should go without saying to never, ever eat food—especially chips or ice cream—directly from the container! Place a specific amount in a small bowl or dish.

Avoid Buffets

When I was in high school, I worked at my aunt and uncle's ice cream business. One of the perks of being an employee was that I could eat ice cream whenever I wanted, especially the mistakes we made while serving the dairy treats to customers. At first, the idea that I could have unlimited access to ice cream seemed incredible—the dream of any teen! Ice cream at your command! Of course, I overate, at least at first.

Over time (and ten pounds later), the thrill wore off and I grew tired of ice cream and ate less. Because of something called sensory-specific satiety, I got tired of eating the same food. Eventually, I had had enough ice cream and preferred to move on to other foods.

In a study on M&Ms at the University of Illinois, the more variety of M&M colors, the more M&Ms people ate.[7] In another study at the same institution, changing the variety of jelly beans prompted people to eat more jelly beans than when their choices were limited. We eat more when there is more variety. If we could snack only on ice cream, we would eventually grow tired of it (but trust me on this, you might pack on quite a few pounds before reaching that point).

However, we have access to a variety of foods. This is why we overeat at buffets. We try a little of this and a little of that. We love the variety, the smells, and the presentation of new foods. If you struggle with your weight, avoid buffets. Instead, order from a menu and limit the variety by ordering one or two items, not a host of appetizers or a family-style meal. Also be aware that the dinnerware and portion size may encourage you to eat more than you really need or want.

Many times I have ordered a pasta dish in an Italian restaurant and been served an immense portion. After eating about a fourth of the dish, I usually have had enough, and have it wrapped up to take home. If I leave it on the table, I end up picking at it because it is in front of me.

You don't want to eat a boring diet, but make sure that plenty of your choices are healthful foods, and that you limit the number and type of high-calorie, low-nutrient options available. Barbara Rolls, PhD, at Penn State University, author of *The Volumetric Weight-Control Plan*, recommends eating low-energy dense foods such as broth-based soups, fresh fruits and vegetables, and high-fiber breakfast cereals to control hunger.[8]

It's also important to introduce food variety to children at an early age, so they experience a number of healthful foods and learn

It Seems Boring, but Read Those Labels!

Dietitians are big on reading labels. But who wants to stand in the grocery store and look at all those ingredients? Most of us don't take the time.

One of the reasons dietitians stress this task is so we know the serving size of what we are eating. Too many people grossly overestimate serving sizes. In my practice at the Center for Eating Disorders, when the dietitians brought out food models that show serving sizes, our clients gasped at how small a true serving size really is.

For example, a serving size of my favorite frozen yogurt is only 170 calories. But according to the label, a serving size is half a cup. Almost no one eats only half a cup. I also usually eat an entire can of soup, while a can is usually considered two servings, not one.

At a YMCA health fair, we gave kids who came to our booth a list of foods and asked them to pick out the serving sizes of several foods, using various props. We asked them to select from a group of items the one that represented a cup of pasta—a tennis ball was the correct answer. Other examples were three ounces of meat (a deck of cards), a slice of bread (an audiocassette tape), and one ounce of cheese (four stacked dice). The children and the adults who played the game with them all overestimated the serving sizes.

Our concept of a serving size is distorted because of the large serving sizes provided by most restaurants. If I thought that a pasta serving in my favorite Italian restaurant was one serving, I would be way off. Usually my plate could feed a family of four! And what is now a kid's meal at most fast-food restaurants was a serving size for adults years ago, according to an article in *The American Journal of Public Health*.[9]

So look at the serving size on the label and be aware of how much you are eating. Pay attention to your internal cues. Eat slowly, chew well, and ask, "Did that amount satisfy my hunger?"

In Japanese, *hara hachi bu* means "eat until you are 80 percent full." And according to studies at Texas Women's University, Okinawans eat less than Americans and eat about half the portion sizes we do.[10] *Hara hachi bu* is a good principle to employ in your own mindset toward eating. Eat until you are 80 percent full. *Press pause* and wait for your stomach and brain to signal fullness.

to eat them. (Remember that children seldom like a new food the first time they try it; they need to sample it several times.) Then by the time they are teenagers, they won't restrict their diets to burgers and fries.

Food variety is a positive thing in terms of food enjoyment and healthful eating. We just have to be careful how much we eat.

Keep the Evidence in Plain Sight

Apparently seeing our leftovers or food wrappers can help us to *not* overeat.

A 2007 Cornell University study[11] was conducted to see how many chicken wings students would eat in a night during a Super Bowl party. The wings were free and students could eat as many as they wanted. However, servers were instructed to leave the bowls with the leftover wing bones on the tables of one group and clear the bowls of chicken bones for another group. As people were eating, some had the evidence (the bones) of how much they ate in front of them, while others did not.

Those who saw the bones in the bowls ate less than those who didn't. The more we see the evidence of what we have eaten—the wrappers, the emptied glasses, the dirty dishes, and so on—the more likely it is that we will eat less.

So when you visit buffets that sweep away the dirty plates while you continue to eat, think about the chicken wing study and ask your waitress to let the plates pile up on the table. It just may save you a few calories!

More Environmental Cues

According to the *Journal of Marketing Research*[12] and Dr. Wansink, author of *Mindless Eating*, a number of other environmental cues also lead to unintentional eating, as follow:

Good deals. We buy more food when we perceive it to be a good deal. Signs such as two for ten dollars and four for a dollar encourages us to pick up those bargains. And we know when we buy more, we tend to eat more.

Bad guessing. We tend to underestimate calories when we approach meals. Typically the bigger the meal, the more our estimates are wrong.[13]

See-through packaging. We are more likely to eat food we have stored in see-through packaging (such as plastic wrap) than food stored in non-see-through packaging (such as aluminum foil).

Our thoughts. The more we like a food, the faster we chew and swallow it; the more we visualize a food, the better our chances of eating it.

Food descriptions. The more we like the description of the food, the more we will buy it and evaluate it as good.

Overall, much in our food environments contributes to unintentional eating. The best thing we can do is be aware of all the ways these environmental factors influence our eating habits. Then we can make modifications that make sense to us, such as downsizing our dinnerware, wrapping leftovers in aluminum foil, monitoring the portion size of foods, and reading labels.

We can focus more on moderation than on abundance, and quality instead of quantity, and enjoy what we do choose to eat. Be aware that your surroundings influence your eating choices. *Press pause* and attend to your environment.

THE PRESS PAUSE PRINCIPLE

Pause to reflect on environmental cues that could be adding extra calories. Do you eat from large plates or drink from short, wide glasses?

Attend to those environmental cues at any given moment. Think about music, variety, smell, and all the other triggers mentioned.

Understand that these cues operate outside of our everyday awareness but that we can bring them to our awareness.

Strategize ways to rearrange your environment or not be tricked by the cues.

Execute changes:
- ▷ Downsize dinnerware.
- ▷ Read labels for portion sizes.
- ▷ Look at the evidence of what you have eaten.
- ▷ Store food out of sight.
- ▷ If you buy big quantities of food, repackage in smaller serving sizes.

PAUSE FOR WISDOM

He who does not mind his belly will hardly mind anything else.

SAMUEL JOHNSON

8

FOOD, MARRIAGE, AND FAMILY

My husband drives me crazy. Actually, he drives me to eat! I am so tired of telling him to pick up after himself. I feel like his servant, constantly picking up his clothes, tools, and personal items that he leaves everywhere. It's not like I don't have enough to do taking care of our four kids. Is it too much to ask him to be more responsible for his things?

One of the least-talked-about reasons for unintentional eating has to do with our interpersonal relationships. It's not that other people make us eat. We are responsible for what we put in our mouths. But our relationships can and do influence our eating. Like the wife speaking above, sometimes we eat because of relationship frustrations. We can also eat in response to relationship conflicts, expectations, and intimacy issues. So you need to attend to relationship issues that may trigger unintentional eating.

In addition, simply being with other people versus eating alone makes a difference in how much we eat. The more we pay attention to how our interpersonal lives cue our eating, the more healthfully we can eat.

The More the Merrier

Eating is a social activity, but eating with even one other person increases your chances of overeating by 35 percent, according to a study by psychologist John de Castro from Sam Houston State University in Huntsville, Texas.[1] Add a group of seven or more to your dining pleasure and you will eat almost twice as much as what you would have by yourself.

When you eat with other people, you are socializing and not paying attention to what or how much you are eating. And when a group of people eat together, usually a variety of food is present, which can contribute to overeating.

Some people find eating with other people to be awkward or tense, and may eat more just to keep themselves occupied and to control anxiety levels. And when you eat with people who eat fast, you tend to speed up your eating to match their pace. So when eating with other people, match your pace to someone who is eating slowly. You can still enjoy the company of others; just focus on the slower eaters.

If you're normally quiet at group meals, try to participate in the conversation. The more you share stories and anecdotes, the less time you'll have to eat.

Tension Leads to Bad Eating Habits

In high school, my friends wanted to eat at my house. We always had tasty home-cooked meals, and dinner hours were lively and full of conversation. This wasn't the case when I visited several of my friends' homes at dinnertime.

At one friend's house, dinner was tense and uncomfortable. The mother was overly focused on manners and proper eating and the dad was harsh and rarely spoke. Another friend's parents began drinking the minute they arrived home. Dinnertime was chaotic and full of commotion.

So consider the atmosphere at your dinner table. Earlier, I talked about the importance of creating a positive atmosphere at mealtimes. One of the ways you accomplish this is by treating people well at the dinner table. If mealtimes are tense and full of conflict, people learn to associate eating with negativity. Let's look at two families, the Joneses and the Smiths.

The Jones family suffers from too much stress, and mealtimes are no exception. The meal is served in a hurry, with people needing to eat quickly and move on to the next activity. Dad discusses the school day with his two teenage children, ending up yelling at one of them for getting poor grades. The younger teen feels caught in the cross fire and eats anxiously to avoid involvement in the conversation. Both children dread dinnertime because of the ongoing tension that never seems to get resolved. Eating together is not an activity this family enjoys. It is the time of day when problems are raised.

The Smiths, however, eat dinner early so no one has to rush off to the next activity. Everyone sits down leisurely to eat and talks about one thing that happened during the day for which they feel grateful. Mealtime conversation is relaxed and upbeat. Meals are a positive point of connection for the entire family. Family members laugh, joke, and encourage one another, and look forward to eating together.

Now, this doesn't mean that the Smiths don't have conflicts or interpersonal issues. They do, but choose to deal with them at other times of the day so they don't associate eating with tension. Mealtimes are times to give thanks and focus on the positive moments of the day. Meals are used to reinforce a sense of belonging and family. This atmosphere provides family members a needed point of contact during their busy day and is a natural platform for relationship building.

Because mealtimes may be one of the few times we actually see family members during our day, it is tempting to use this time to complain and focus on problems. But think of how pleasant it would be for mealtimes to become a place of sanctuary instead of stress.

And while we relax around the table, it's a good idea to compliment the cook or cooks! Praise and gratitude go a long way when it comes to building positive relationships. Use mealtimes to strengthen intimate connections, not tear them down.

Consider Your Expectations

We all come to relationships with certain expectations, whether we know it or not. Expectations develop based on our experiences with others, especially people we are close to. If we grew up in a home where people were dependable, we carry that expectation into our relationships with other people—we expect them to be dependable as well. If we grew up in a home where people were dishonest, we tend to approach our relationships expecting people to be dishonest.

Problems emerge when our expectations don't match up to our reality. We expect things of people and they don't deliver. When this happens, we can respond in one of two ways: accept it or become upset. Obviously, we need to realize that people won't always meet our expectations. However, when you are disappointed or hurt, don't use food to cope with those feelings.

Mary was upset when her husband, Tyler, spent evenings with his buddies; she spent her evenings alone, filling her loneliness with food. Tyler thought it was normal to go out with his friends once a week, and was frustrated that Mary gave him a hard time about what he considered normal, healthy behavior.

The problem here is expectations. Mary expected Tyler to devote all his free time to her. Tyler expected to have certain outings without his wife while married. The couple needed to negotiate these differing expectations around the use of free time. Once they agreed to what both considered reasonable expectations, Mary's unintentional eating diminished.

Notice how Mary and Tyler dealt with their expectations. First they had to acknowledge them, then they negotiated them. One of the biggest problems I see in therapy is that people are not even aware of their expectations. They don't *press pause* and ask, *What are my expectations for this relationship, for my family?* Yet this is very important to prevent unintentional eating.

When our expectations include the need for people to be perfect, to do things our way, to anticipate our every need or to complete us, we have problems and may eat our way through disappointment. Let's look at how these issues influence our eating.

Perfectionism

A perfectionist may obsess with food because he or she is anxious most of the time. "My children must be model children and I can't allow myself to make a mistake," says one perfectionist. "It's exhausting to live like this but if I relax for even a moment, I'm afraid something will go wrong. The one place I'm not perfect is with food. I try to control every bite that goes into my mouth, but I can't. And because of this, I feel guilty all the time."

At the heart of a perfectionist are self-defeating thoughts fueled by unrealistic expectations. Perfectionists believe their worth is based on what they do and what they accomplish. They don't understand unconditional love. Mistakes mean failure. The constant cycle to achieve perfection leads to feelings of self-defeat and failure. These negative feelings can prompt unintentional eating.

The fix involves setting realistic goals, understanding that worth is not based on accomplishments, allowing yourself to make mistakes, and learning to focus more on the present rather than the end goal.

Perfectionism is bondage that often translates to food and eating. It leads to body dissatisfaction and can lead to eating disorders. If you struggle with perfectionism, begin to evaluate your expectations. Once you identify your thoughts, you'll need to renegotiate those expectations.

The Land Mines of Expectations

Jerry thought it was reasonable for his stay-at-home wife, Pamela, to have dinner on the table when he came home, and thinks she should make this a priority. Pamela is frustrated that Jerry doesn't understand the demands of three small children and her part-time work at home. She thinks his expectations are unrealistic and she wants more understanding and flexibility from him.

Jerry is saying, *Do it my way,* regardless of Pamela's problems in trying to accommodate him. This type of control is often the basis of marital problems. If you won't negotiate expectations and be flexible, problems emerge. As a response to Jerry's inflexible expectation concerning dinner, Pamela began to pick at food during the day and mindlessly eat.

To get control of her eating, Pamela had to revisit this expectation with Jerry. She talked about the logistics of the problem in getting dinner on the table and asked Jerry to help her problem-solve. He did and offered to help her some nights. Jerry became more flexible when he realized that Pamela's failure to meet his expectations was not a sign of an uncaring wife. He mistakenly believed that if she loved him, she would have dinner on the table. When he was a boy, he actually heard his dad say this to his mom. But in Jerry's family today, Pamela's difficulty in preparing dinner had nothing to do with love. It was more about the busyness of her life. Once Jerry recognized this, he relaxed and was helpful.

Seeking Completion

People often come into relationships with the idea that someone else will complete them and make them whole. They see their lives like a puzzle with a piece missing that someone else will supply. This expectation is bound to cause problems, including overeating.

When Naomi married Mark, she was rebounding from a troubled relationship with a man who was verbally abusive. Naomi's relationship with her father was distant and cold. She never felt the love and affection she desperately wanted from her dad. As a result, she tried to find men who could make up for the hole she felt in her heart.

When she started dating Mark, he was attentive and loving. But when they married, he became more like her father—distant and cold.

As Naomi sat in the therapy office, she wondered how she could have misjudged Mark and other men so dramatically. "I really thought Mark was different from the others. He seemed so caring and attentive."

Yet the courtship with Mark was short. What Naomi didn't know was that Mark had a history of going after women, sweeping them off their feet, and then dumping them. Mark was in it for the excitement of the chase. When the chase was over, he lost interest.

The more Naomi talked about their dating history, the more she realized that she had been the one pushing marriage. Her motivation was to find a man who gave her the love her father could not. She was looking for a man to complete her rather than grieving the loss of an emotionally cold father. Now she found herself mindlessly eating to cope with the familiar feeling of emotional distance, which she felt with Mark.

Naomi was able to give up mindless eating when she grieved the loss of an intimate relationship with her father and began addressing the lack of emotional intimacy in her marriage.

When we look to other people to complete us, we will be disappointed. Rather than seeking others to make up for what we are missing, we must grieve what we didn't get as a loss. Then we grow and can approach our new relationships in a healthier way.

The Pressures of Being a Parent

Responsibilities associated with marriage and raising a family can become routine and boring at times. It's no fun to change diapers, clean house, run errands, or pay bills. These mundane tasks can lead to the refrigerator. The trick is not to use food to relieve boredom or routine.

Keisha had two small children and was a stay-at-home mom. She loved her children, but she was bored and physically exhausted; she craved adult conversation and time alone. "I know this is just a season in my life, but I suspect I eat because I feel bored a lot," she said.

We can all appreciate Keisha's honesty. She was saying what many women feel but don't express. Keisha is a great mom who just needs balance in her life. Fortunately, Keisha found an easy fix. She scheduled playdates with children whose parents agreed to talk about subjects other than kids. This way, she could take her kids on outings and enjoy adult company and conversation with other moms.

Keisha also joined a Mothers Day Out program for preschool children at a local church. She used this time one morning a week to run errands and do things that fulfilled her as a person. Sometimes it was reading a book, window shopping, or having coffee at a local café. Most often, she met a friend just to talk and catch up. But the short time she spent energizing herself was enough to revitalize her for family duties. She simply needed a little balance between meeting the constant needs of others and her own needs.

Once Keisha felt less drained of personal energy, she stopped using food to cope with family stress. And the small amount of time she took for herself each week lessened the boredom. She had something to look forward to and no longer needed food as a diversion from boredom.

Starving for Intimacy

Perhaps the most common marital issue I see is eating as a replacement for love and affection. Because food is associated with caring and affection, when intimacy in an important relationship is missing, food can become the substitute.

Greg and his wife haven't been intimate for months, and he misses spending time alone with her. When they do have sex, it's hurried and not passionate. He misses romance in his life, and compensates by frequently grabbing food from the fridge.

For Greg, food is replacing intimacy. The problem is that food doesn't work very well to solve the intimacy problem. The solution to end his unintentional eating is to attend to Greg's wish to be more intimate with his wife.

Because Greg recognized the connection between lost intimacy and eating, he was able to do something about it. He and his wife are now spending more time together. They instituted a date night once a week and have made a conscious effort to be more affectionate with each other during their week. They greet each other with a kiss, hold hands, cuddle on the couch, and make time for sex.

Gaining Weight to Protect Yourself

Some people eat to gain weight to protect themselves from their own sexual feelings or the sexual advances of others. The source of the eating can vary, but the basic reasoning is the same.

To protect against abuse. Jana was date raped when she was a teenager. On some level Jana believes that her thinness and attractiveness caused this man to rape her, and now she eats mindlessly to keep a protective layer of fat on her body.

Only when Jana faces her fears and loses the misplaced guilt and shame will she be able to stop "protecting" herself with eating. As Jana faces the loss of control she experienced when raped, she will eventually regain control over eating.

To keep from cheating. Married for ten years, Alexis's marriage felt empty and unfulfilling. She and her husband had grown apart. Alexis, a child of divorce, did not want to bring divorce into her family. She wanted her children to grow up with both parents. She felt stuck and used food as a coping strategy to keep her own sexual impulses at bay. Her extra weight kept her from cheating on her husband.

Once Alexis became aware that her unintentional eating was a protection from sexually acting out, she could make the choice of facing the emotional distance in her marriage or continue overeating as a protective mechanism.

Alexis chose to work on her marriage and began marital therapy. She found she still had feelings of affection for her husband, and they solved their unhappy feelings. As a result, Alexis no longer used food to keep her sexual impulses at bay. Her sex life became satisfied in the marriage.

To keep a spouse at bay. Debbie was no longer interested in having sex with her husband, and was extremely uncomfortable talking to her husband about sex. When she was growing up, any discussion about sex was taboo. When she married, this didn't change. As the years passed, this couple's sex life had greatly deteriorated and neither one of them confronted the problem. Debbie's solution was to eat to gain weight and turn off her husband sexually. Then she could justify the rejection and not confront the underlying problem of a boring sex life.

The fix involved uncomfortable conversations about the couple's sex life. Both had to learn to tolerate these uncomfortable feelings and push through to get answers. Once they did, unintentional eating to create distance was no longer necessary.

Look at how you may use eating to handle intimacy issues. Think about what relationship issues may lead you to unintentionally eat. Attend to conflicts, problems, and sources of interpersonal stress. See a therapist if you need help. As you attend to your relationships, you just might find a trigger for unintentional eating.

THE PRESS PAUSE PRINCIPLE

Plan in your heart to think about your relationships.

Attend to the number of people with whom you eat, the setting, and any relationship conflicts, issues, stresses, or problems that may trigger unintentional eating.

Understand the importance that relationships play in our unconscious eating and how expectations, frustrations, conflicts, and lack of intimacy can trigger overeating.

Strategize by identifying relationship issues and the triggers that may lead to eating.

Execute changes:
- ▷ Be mindful when eating with other people, pace yourself with the slower eaters at a table, and interact with other diners.
- ▷ Identify relationship expectations. Are they reasonable? If not, begin to think about what would be reasonable.
- ▷ Identify specific issues of intimacy that may be contributing to unintentional eating and work on those issues. You may need to see a counselor for help.

PAUSE FOR WISDOM

One cannot think well, love well, sleep well,
if one has not dined well.

VIRGINIA WOOLF

PART THREE

UNDERSTAND

Once you pause and attend to the moment, you can increase your understanding of what is happening to your body, soul, and spirit. To understand *why* we do what we do is important for any sustained change. Understanding our relationship with food helps us focus on what we need to change.

To develop a positive relationship with food and become more intentional in our eating, we have to look at what interferes with these goals. What gets in our way of seeing and using food in positive ways? Why do we want to make changes in our relationship with food but often fail at doing so? Why do we have good intentions but so often fail to live differently? Are you emotionally or spiritually hungry and using food to satisfy these hungers? Are your thoughts about food self-judgmental and negative, leading you to feel bad about yourself and eat more? The answers to such questions will help us get to the root of why we do what we do.

The better you understand your current relationship with food and eating, the easier it will be to make changes. This type of understanding will help you know why you eat for unintended reasons. And understanding often brings compassion to the eating struggle, allowing you to begin making changes.

This section is about understanding emotions, thoughts, and spiritual cravings that lead to unintentional eating. And when we understand the power of our thoughts in determining our actions, we can strategize ways to renew our minds and enjoy eating.

9

FEASTING ON EMOTIONS

There is a definite connection between food and mood. Whether we are reeling from a divorce, struggling with a migraine, visiting the unemployment line, or happy because a raise came though, we often use food as a release. We use it to soothe a bad feeling, celebrate a good one, or avoid a feeling altogether.

Even dealing with daily hassles such as commuter traffic, a late appointment, or an unscheduled visit from your nosy aunt can drive you to the refrigerator or prompt you to bake a batch of chocolate chip cookies.

Both adults and children eat in response to happy and uncomfortable feelings. It is a learned behavior that we either model from others or discover on our own. We hurt, we eat, and then feel better, or we are happy and eat to celebrate. The cycle is repeated. Once emotional eating becomes habitual, we overeat without thinking or understanding why we put food in our mouths. We need to understand the connection between emotions and food so we can make changes.

Food works to offset emotions and unpleasant feelings more than we'd like to believe. I estimate that 75 percent of the overeating I've seen in my practice is emotionally based. To stop unintentional and hurried eating, understanding emotional hunger is critical.

The Connection Between Food and Emotions

Emotional eating keeps us from feeling bad for the moment or extends happy feelings a bit longer. But it also keeps us stuck when it comes to losing weight or maintaining our weight. Food can be used like a drug. It can medicate, numb, distract, and help us escape emotional pain.

We need to explore the ways our emotions can cause us to overeat. Getting to the root of why we eat is critical to defeating unhealthy eating. To do so requires a better understanding of our emotional lives. Once we understand the connection between food and mood, it is possible to learn how to better handle our emotional states without turning to food.

Press pause and identify which emotions you feel or are attempting not to feel and why. Are you happy, angry, bored, tired, sad, or

Why We Eat What We Eat

Let's look at what research tells us about our relationship with food, and how mood affects our cravings and the amount of food we eat.

When happy, we tend to choose foods that have more nutritional value than the foods chosen when we are sad or down, says Brian Wansink, PhD, the food marketing psychologist at Cornell University and executive director of the USDA's Center for Nutrition Policy and Promotion. When we want to celebrate a raise, the birth of a child, or our son's piano recital, we reward ourselves with food, but choose foods such as pizza or steak versus ice cream and cookies.

Some foods actually help boost our moods, according to studies published in *Psychopharmacology* and *Archives internationales de pharmacodynamie et de thérapie*.[1] Chocolate-covered almonds provide a two-part boost: the almonds help increase dopamine levels and the chocolate stimulates serotonin. Both of these brain chemicals improve our mood by stimulating these mood-enhancing neurotransmitters in the brain. Of course, remember to eat chocolate-covered almonds in moderation!

People eat when happy, lonely, anxious, tired, sad, and angry. According to a survey by Dr. Wansink,[2] people turned to comfort food 86 percent of the time when happy, 74 percent of the time for reward, 52 percent of the time in response to boredom, 39 percent of the time for depression, and 39 percent of the time for loneliness.

Women choose foods based on their emotional needs, while men reach for comfort foods when they are happy. Studies cited in the *Journal of Psychology*[3] show that people more often consume healthful foods when experiencing positive emotions, and unhealthful foods when experiencing negative emotions. We eat more when experiencing either positive or negative emotions, and anger and joy influence eating more than fear and sadness, according to studies cited in *Appetite*.[4]

And parents model eating habits for their children: a Dutch study reported in *Appetite*[5] found a connection between parents who were emotional eaters and teens who did the same. The bottom line is that mood affects our cravings and the amount of food we eat.

lonely? Stop and ask, *What would I be feeling if I wasn't eating this food?*

How We Try to Fix Things with Food

The problem with using food as a fix for emotional states is that once the food is consumed, emotions resurface. Food is only a temporary fix. Let's look at how two people use food to numb their feelings and to help distract them from problems.

Upset over a breakup with her boyfriend, Whitney decided not to be alone, at least for the evening. She knew that if she returned to her apartment, she would sit in front of the television, eat, and feel sorry for herself. So she texted three of her girlfriends and asked them to meet her for dinner at a local hot spot.

At the restaurant, the women greeted one another and ordered appetizers and drinks. The conversation quickly became engaging. Without realizing it, Whitney had devoured buffalo wings, chicken fingers, and nachos before the meal ever began. As the women continued to wallow over relationship woes, they ordered meals, followed by a round of hot fudge sundaes. Whitney felt relieved. The food and friendships distracted her from the hurt she felt inside. She didn't have to think about the loss of her relationship. Food temporarily numbed any feelings of loss. What she didn't realize is that she could have enjoyed the companionship and comfort of her friends *without* overindulging as she did.

One Saturday, the guys invited Ron over to watch college football and get away from the house for a few hours. Beer, pizza, chips, and cookies were spread out on the bar, and Ron ate several helpings. It seems Ron and his wife fight about everything, but for the time being he put the problems with his wife out of his mind. The game was a welcomed distraction.

The guys had a great time screaming and yelling at the teams. The experience reminded Ron of his carefree single days. However, without thinking, Ron ate and drank more than he intended. Food distracted him from the intimacy problems he faced with his wife. After the game, Ron had to go home and face the problems in his marriage—with an overfull belly.

Whitney and Ron engaged in a form of social emotional eating. It happens all the time. Getting together with friends or family when we are upset, anxious, worried, or even happy makes us feel better, at least for the moment. We don't have to think about our problems or we can release a happy emotion through food.

Food can distract us from the issues at hand. It eases our hurt and emotional pain. It numbs our senses and provides temporary pleasure.

But crying over a nightmare date with a tub of ice cream and trying not to remember the hurtful words of a spouse by munching on goodies are not productive ways to deal with emotions. They don't solve the problem, and they make us feel worse afterward. We need to learn how to cope with our emotions in healthy ways—without food.

Eating Ourselves Happy

Robert was excited. After months of tedious practice, he had performed well at his piano recital. He had worked hard at memorizing a difficult piece and his performance reflected well on that effort. Robert's teacher beamed as his family and friends congratulated him on a job well done. Robert almost felt high from the excitement and wanted to celebrate.

His family suggested they go out to eat and celebrate with a big dinner. The meal included numerous appetizers before the steaks arrived at the table. After dining with delight and feeling overly full and sleepy, the family decided to call it a night. Robert wanted to savor the moment and didn't want the night to end. It felt so good to have accomplished what he did. He was happy.

In another example, Rick was elated that he finally received a much deserved raise. Sitting in his office with check in hand, he felt happy. The feeling felt so good that he took a break to reward himself with a big batch of hot wings from the deli next door.

Robert and Rick were rewarding themselves with food—releasing happiness through food.

It's wonderful to reward ourselves for jobs well done or to celebrate happy events; it's not wonderful if food is the only way we can express happiness, or if we eat mindlessly on these happy occasions.

Eating to Hide from Pain

Jennifer was a shy child who never had many friends in her grade-school class. When her classmates arranged playdates, Jennifer was left out. She couldn't invite classmates to her house because they might somehow learn that her father sexually abused her. And he told her that if she ever told anyone, they would hate her.

Jennifer felt trapped. She couldn't talk about what was happening in her life. She felt dirty and ashamed but saw no way out. To endure the regular sexual abuse, Jennifer would focus her mind on the clouds outside her bedroom window and try to imagine them as cotton candy and lollipops. It was the only way she could tolerate the violation being done to her. As she grew, food became her friend and sanctuary. She imagined food whenever she felt emotional pain and ate to escape that pain. Eventually she hit 340 pounds.

Children like Jennifer who are traumatized by abuse often use food to cover the emotional pain or to distract them from ongoing abuse. Other children are teased and mocked because they look a certain way, aren't smart enough, or don't fit in with the group. Food becomes their way to cope with the hurt of rejection. Food doesn't reject you. It is always available, tastes good, and never talks back. It is a good companion when others are not. It fills a void for children who are neglected or suffer loss and don't have the emotional support of others.

Eating to Gain Control

I've worked with children who hide food under their beds. At night, when their parents fight, drink, or are out of control, the hidden food stash is a source of comfort. They eat to calm down, to soothe themselves, or to feel pleasure. Hiding food gives them control over something. They can have food when they want or need it.

Several children I've counseled sneaked food as a way to deal with power issues in their families. They felt their parents were too rigid and demanding and that hiding food was their way of having some control. Sneaking food was an act of independence or rebellion.

These families had to work on issues of autonomy and authority. Parents who were too demanding of their children needed to be less rigid and more emotionally sensitive in order to develop their children's autonomy in healthy ways. When the parents developed more flexibility and sensitivity to the needs of their children, sneaking food was no longer needed.

A study of first graders reported in *Pediatrics*[6] showed that extremely strict and controlling parents had a higher rate of overweight kids than those who set limits and consequences but were warm and encouraging. Permissive and neglectful styles of parenting also increased the risk for overweight children.

Furthermore, children brought up in homes with overly strict parents don't learn to eat based on hunger and fullness cues.[7] These parents tend to use food as a reward or restrict the kind or amount of food that the child can eat. Eating behind a parent's back can be a reaction to excessive control. Of course, indulging kids doesn't help them learn to set limits and attend to the cues of their bodies. The best approach is to be authoritative—warm and encouraging with limits and structure.

Adults who tackle their emotional eating habits help their children learn better ways of coping. So if you need incentive to *press pause* and identify why you eat, here it is—you can stop the pattern of emotional eating in your home.

Eating for Loneliness and Boredom

Matthew was a bright and accomplished man who worked hard. While he could produce an event with ease, he fought his weight. Diet after diet failed and his weight remained high. Nothing he tried seemed to work until he came to therapy.

He learned that food was a distraction from the long, boring hours of work. It gave him pleasure when bored. It kept him company and prevented him from thinking too long about the emotional emptiness of his life.

He was completely devoted to his career, having long ago given up on the possibility of love, children, or even friendships. When they didn't come, he poured himself into work and never took the time to develop other parts of his life. His accomplishments reinforced his efforts.

At events that required small talk, he was socially anxious. Holidays were painful reminders of his decision to make work his top priority. Without work, he had little to think about. He stopped talking to his family regularly because he was too busy and wanted to avoid questions about his free time. He tried not to think about the emptiness he often felt and filled it with food.

Matthew knew other single people his age who allowed people into their lives and developed social and spiritual lives apart from their careers. He realized it wasn't too late to make changes, and that food could no longer be his distraction, friend, and partner.

For most of his adult life, he had used food to fill loneliness, and trained himself not to think about the pain he experienced. The thought of not distracting himself from reality frightened him. He knew his anxiety would rise if he gave up the familiar. But he was ready to try.

His first step was to find an interest apart from work. His father had been an avid seaman who taught him to love the water, so he signed up for a beginning sailing class.

The first night of class was overwhelming. He felt anxious, awkward, and uncomfortable making small talk with strangers. He wanted to run and eat but resisted. *Just stick it out. It will get better,* he reminded himself. *I'm doing something I don't feel competent doing. It should make me feel anxious. My therapist says this isn't bad.*

Week by week the anxiety he felt improved, and he also found a church to attend. Gradually, with patience and persistence, he replaced the emptiness of his life with friendships and spiritual meaning. It wasn't easy and the temptation to use food as friend and distraction was compelling. But with his faith and community, he felt strong.

How do you know if you are using food as a distraction from boredom or loneliness? Think about your losses—the loss of expectation, of health, of dreams, or relationships:

- Are you disappointed in your career?
- Have you given up on a dream to have a career that excites you?
- Are you fighting an ailment or setback, and feeling that life isn't fair?
- Is your marriage struggling?
- Have you grieved your losses and moved forward or are you stuck in feelings of anger, denial, or sadness?

Eating for Anxiety

Do you think you would be more social if you dropped twenty pounds? But perhaps your discomfort with social situations has less to do with weight and more to do with the anxiety you feel around others. Weight can be an easy excuse to hide behind.

Carol was convinced that if she dropped a significant amount of weight, she would begin dating and eventually marry. In her mind, it was all about the weight. I didn't agree. She was socially anxious and hard on men, because of the difficult relationship she had with her father. Losing weight might boost her confidence but wouldn't address the social anxiety she felt or the anger she carried toward men. And both of those issues blocked her ability to form an intimate relationship. The weight was an excuse to avoid taking an honest look at her life.

Social situations can trigger anxiety if you don't feel comfortable in your own skin. You may hover by the food table at a social event to calm down or eat in response to nervous energy. Or you may eat to fit in or eat because others upset you and you don't know how to handle those feelings. Eating can become a nervous habit like cracking knuckles or pacing.

Monica used food to calm her jitters. She was a first-time mom who described her childhood as very unhappy and problematic; she feared she would re-create that unhappiness for her own child. To cope with her anxious parenting, she grazed on food all day.

Anxious feelings can trigger urges to eat. Food can soothe and calm you down temporarily. You must learn to manage those anxious feelings and not use food this way. Whenever you have the urge to eat, write down the feeling you are having. When you feel anxious, turn to a list of things you can do instead of eat:

▸ Call a friend.
▸ Take a nap.

- ▸ Drink a glass of water.
- ▸ Walk around the block.
- ▸ Meditate.
- ▸ Clean your house.
- ▸ Play with your pet.

Anything that breaks the cycle of using food to calm down is worth a try as long as it isn't another addiction. (Turn to the suggestions in chapter 12 on managing emotions.)

Some people need therapy to work on issues that trigger anxiety. In my years of practice, I have often found that anxiety was tied to unexpected loss and failure to grieve, and often triggered by faulty thinking. Whatever the source of your anxiety, it takes courage to get at the root, but the effort will be worth it. Once you face the issue you've been avoiding and work through it, it will no longer hold power over you.

Others may have to work on anxiety and fears related to trusting people and including them in their lives. Perhaps you have been betrayed, abandoned, rejected, or left to fend for yourself. Letting other people into your intimate life can be frightening.

Still others may need to confront anxiety that results from spiritual emptiness. This is an emptiness that cannot be filled by your own efforts. When we try to do everything on our own, we can become increasingly more anxious and worried. In the New Testament of the Bible, Jesus tells us to not worry or become anxious because he watches and cares for us. If we believe in a supernatural partnership with One who is mindful of us and supplies our daily needs, worry takes a backseat.

A personal, authentic relationship with God is the only way to fill that spiritual void, which will be discussed in a later chapter. The first step is always to surrender your anxiety to God and allow him to be in charge of your life. The promised benefits are peace, rest, and the ability to not be anxious.

Eating Because You're Tired

It has been a rough day and you are exhausted. You come home. The kids are crying, your spouse unloads all the problems of the day, and you just want to escape. Instead, you make a beeline for the refrigerator, take snacks to the couch, and flop down in front of the television.

Our exhausted bodies want fuel for energy, so we load up. And when we are tired, we aren't as disciplined about the amount and nutritional value of our food choices. It's easy to reach for the chips and dip and crunch our way to relaxation.

Studies suggest that when we eat in response to feeling tired, we tend to overeat.[8] Dr. Allan Rechtschaffen, director of the Sleep Research Laboratory at the University of Chicago, tells us that people who don't get enough sleep tend to increase their calories by 10 to 15 percent over what they need. Because core-body temperature goes down when we are sleep deprived, eating is a way to compensate for that lost heat energy.

It doesn't take much to tire us out. We often push ourselves beyond reasonable limits because we have so much to do and so little time to do it. The result is chronic tiredness. Sometimes we eat just to keep going. Food gives us that energy boost to make it through a sleepy morning, a long afternoon, or an exhausting evening. But the burst of energy is short-lived. A good nap or getting to bed on time usually helps. Both body and mind function best when we are well rested.

Workaholic Ann learned this the hard way. Her schedule left her little time to rest or sleep. Her day began at 5:00 a.m. Grabbing food on the way out the door, Ann caught the 6:30 a.m. train into the city. She usually stayed at the office until 6:00 or 7:00 every night before catching the 8:00 train home. By the time she made a quick dinner and worked on projects at her home computer, she rarely made it to bed before 1:00 a.m.

After six months of this schedule, Ann was exhausted and gaining weight. Throughout the day and night, she snacked—usually on convenience and prepared foods—to stay awake and get things done. What she needed to do was get more sleep, eat a well-balanced diet, and establish working hours with limits. Ann's goal is now to be in bed by 11:00 every night. For Ann, a lack of sleep triggered overeating. Once she realized this and made changes, her weight stabilized.

Joyce Walsleben, a registered nurse and director of the Sleep Disorders Center at New York University School of Medicine, likens a person who lacks sleep to a musician who plays out of tune in a symphony. Without sleep, we just don't do our best. As simple as it sounds, we need to make more time for sleep.

Bedtime rituals do help prepare us for sleep. Experiment with different routines to see what works for you. For some people soothing music puts them to sleep. Others like to soak in a hot bath, read, or watch television before bed. Avoid caffeine at night, and move your glow-in-the-dark clock away from your line of sight so that you aren't looking at it all night long. Relax and clear your mind. Prayer is great for refocusing on the blessings of the day and renewing your hope for tomorrow.

Eating from Guilt and Shame

Guilt is a natural response to doing something wrong. We should feel guilty when we commit a crime, treat someone poorly, or say hateful things. Guilt is a feeling of remorse that hopefully motivates us to correct our behavior.

In my work with eating disorders, I often see a strong connection between guilt and eating. Guilt becomes more than the natural response to doing something wrong. It is associated with not being perfect, not measuring up, and not pleasing all people at all times. In these cases, guilt becomes the inability to forgive oneself for not measuring up to some perceived standard, usually unrealistic. When this happens you can feel depressed, anxious, or even angry. To cope with the guilt, you turn to food, then, having binged or compulsively overeaten, you feel guilty and the cycle repeats.

Kate constantly tried to please everyone in her life. When, after much thought, she confronted a friend about a problem, he reacted negatively. Kate then felt guilty for upsetting her friend and binged on food. Kate's guilt was misplaced. She committed no offense. In fact, she acted like a true friend, confronting an issue before it became more of a problem.

Shame also triggers eating. Women and men who have been raped, abused, or traumatized in some way may feel it is their fault. When this happens, they may resort to eating as a way to cover up or hide feelings of shame.

Shame implies that you, as a person, are bad, but isn't tied to perceived wrongdoing as guilt is. Shame comes from being humiliated, teased, threatened, physically hurt, or punished and leads to feelings of worthlessness.

Robin felt shame about her body, and she felt she couldn't physically measure up to images she saw of women in the media. She also felt guilt from an extramarital affair she had and couldn't get thoughts of her "badness" out of her head. Though she'd confessed her wrongdoing and intellectually knew she was forgiven, she couldn't shake the feelings of shame. She felt dirty and worthless and she ate in response to those feelings.

Therapy had to address her thoughts of shame and guilt, which were keeping her stuck and not allowing her to move forward with her life. Yes, the affair was serious and wrong but to continue to beat herself up over something she recognized as wrong was not helping her mental health. She needed the help of a therapist to realize she was no longer condemned for what she had done. Robin believed a lie—she was too bad to be forgiven. She didn't understand the truth about God. When we confess our wrongdoings, God is always faithful to forgive us and wipe our mistakes clean. Healing came when she could accept the forgiveness she was offered by God and learned to forgive herself for her mistakes. She was then able to let go of her shame and guilt, and her urges to binge subsided.

Eating for Anger

Have you ever stuffed your mouth with food rather than expressed anger? Perhaps you were so mad at your boss that you left your desk and made a beeline for the vending machine. Or you had an argument with your spouse and raided the refrigerator. Maybe you ended an angry phone conversation with your mother and drove to the 7-Eleven for some goodies.

Anger is one of the easiest emotions to eat your way through, especially for women who don't like to even acknowledge that they get angry. Research at the University of London suggests that food can be used to medicate strong emotions such as anger.[9]

Amanda learned at an early age to suppress her anger with food. She and her three sisters were told to keep their angry emotions within and pretend everything was fine. But everything wasn't fine and Amanda needed an outlet—eating.

When we don't deal with anger, we may use food to distract us or calm us down. Don uses food to calm himself when angry. His temper easily flares and he knows that he often scares his children because of his quick fuse. So Don resorts to eating as a way to simmer down. His motivation is good—he doesn't want to frighten people. But his strategy is causing other problems: his belly is growing and his anger isn't abating.

Anger can also remain unresolved. When this happens, you might not know that you are eating your way through anger. Are you angry at your boss, your spouse, your friend, your neighbor, a relative? Has that anger simmered for a long time and have you developed the habit of eating and not dealing with the issues at hand? If so, you must forgive and let go of offenses before you will get your eating under control. There are no shortcuts to dealing with anger. The best strategy is to express it in a manner that is healthy and try to resolve the issue. Follow the anger guidelines in chapter 12, or seek help from a therapist.

The point is to know that anger is an eating trigger. Track your emotions to understand your urges to eat. See if you can identify anger triggers. Some of you may have to begin by acknowledging the fact that you get angry. Anger is not wrong, but must be expressed in safe and appropriate ways. So don't suppress anger or pretend it isn't a part of life. Learn to express it properly and move on with life.

Eating for Sadness

Kristen came to me because she was binge eating. She, like many troubled teen girls, also cuts herself to relieve the stress and emotional pain she feels. Stress from school, peers, and her family combined with a media-driven culture have thrown Kristen into such turmoil that harming her body is one way she finds momentary relief. Kristen is not suicidal. She is looking for a way to manage her pain. Self-punishment seems like a workable strategy.

When Kristen tries to stop cutting, she binges on food. Both the bingeing and the cutting are ways she tries to manage her emotional sadness. At times, she would rather feel pain than nothing. When she chooses not to self-injure and to feel pain, she is sad and fills up with food. Then she feels guilty and shameful and tries to stop cutting as well as bingeing.

The root of both of these behaviors is an incredible sadness Kristen feels in her family. There are many demands on Kristen but very little emotional connection. When she came to therapy, she wasn't able to identify this sadness at first. She just knew she felt bad and empty and wanted those feelings to stop. Now Kristen is learning to address her sadness.

Many people drown their sorrows in a bowl of chocolate chip ice cream, a bag of chips, or a steak dinner. They use food to distract them from the sorrow they feel. Food takes them away and helps them feel something good, not sad. It brings momentary pleasure. In Kristen's case, food wasn't enough and her desperation for connection led her to alternate between bingeing and self-injury.

What is important to think about is how you react to sadness and depression. If you eat in response to sadness, you must identify those triggers and work on your mood (turn to chapter 12). Sadness that is prolonged can turn into depression. Depression affects people differently but is treatable and doesn't have to be a trigger for eating or overeating. If your sadness persists, see your physician or a licensed mental health provider for depression treatment.

Identify Emotional Eating and Your Emotional Triggers

It is not difficult to recognize the signs of emotional eating. If it's not a mealtime, ask yourself if you are truly hungry whenever you want to eat, and think about why you are eating. Remember the difference between physical and emotional hungers outlined in chapter 3? If you aren't physically hungry and continue to obsess about food, something emotional is likely at the root.

Emotional eating includes the following:

- ▶ Impulsive eating
- ▶ Binge eating
- ▶ Feeling out of control
- ▶ Eating past feeling full
- ▶ Eating in private so no one will see you
- ▶ Hiding food
- ▶ Eating fast
- ▶ Feeling guilty or remorseful afterward

The easiest way to begin breaking old eating patterns is to keep a short eating diary. Follow the example below. Track what you feel when you have an urge to eat that is not based in physical hunger. Here are some sample entries:

EATING DIARY

TIME OF DAY	3:00 p.m.
SITUATION	Bonus at work
EMOTION	Elated
FOOD	Splurged on chicken wings
TIME OF DAY	5:00 p.m.
SITUATION	Did poorly on a project
EMOTION	Depressed
FOOD	Wanted to eat ice cream
TIME OF DAY	7:00 p.m.
SITUATION	Long day
EMOTION	Tired
FOOD	Ate half a bag of chips and the entire container of dip

Hold on to this diary because we are going to add more to it in the next chapter. For now, just understand how your emotions are connected to food. We'll tackle our thoughts later.

How to Deal with Emotional Eating

When trying to break any bad habit, it helps to focus on the present and not get worked up about the past. If you've eaten mindlessly in the past, let it go and focus on what you can do right now to make a difference. You aren't a victim. You can learn to be mindful and focus your attention on what is happening. When you do, observe your feelings without judging them as good or bad. Accept whatever feeling comes with the urge to eat. Write it down and just observe it at this point. Over time, you will probably notice a pattern. Certain emotions trigger the urge to eat, as do certain times of the day, environmental cues, and thoughts.

Food can be used to distract us from loneliness, boredom, and emotional emptiness. Whether it is the choices we've made, the lack of control we've had, or our unwillingness to move out of our comfort zone, food fills a void and provides a service. It keeps us stuck in the familiar. But we have the choice not to stay stuck once we understand how we use food to cope.

When food becomes a friend or a distraction, we have to be willing to replace it with something of equal or greater meaning. For many of us, that requires engaging with people, building community, and connecting to the power of faith.

It also means confronting people and events that are uncomfortable or even painful. Eating is easier than confronting the loss of expectations. Food can distract us from the pain and anxiety related to loss, and can temporarily fill that empty place. But in the long run, food can't do what you need it to do without negative consequences. Furthermore, food can't give you what people or a rich spiritual life can. So emptiness is ultimately about surrender—surrendering to the power food has over you.

Once you recognize what emotional eating is, *press pause* and identify what emotion has triggered the urge to eat. What are you feeling? What happened to set you off?

Instead of reaching for food as a way to extend the good feeling, do something else to enjoy those happy feelings:

1. Be grateful and count your blessings. When something good happens to you, enjoy the moment and give thanks.
2. Express your feelings of happiness verbally and in writing.
3. Pray and meditate; enrich your spiritual life.
4. Reach out to others. Happiness can be infectious. Connect with friends and family but not necessarily over food.

Enjoy happy feelings, but don't depend on them or expect them to stay with you at all times. Look inward and seek ways to move beyond happiness to states of contentment and peace. Instead of reaching for food to extend happiness, learn to be content in all things.

Once you are aware of which emotions trigger your eating and when, you can make changes to break the cycle. It will require a *pause*—plan, awareness, understanding, strategy, and execution of changes—but you can do it.

THE PRESS PAUSE PRINCIPLE

Plan in your heart to understand emotional hunger.

Attend to your emotional state when eating: What are you feeling?

Understand which emotions lead to eating when not hungry.

Strategize to track those emotions in an eating diary and determine which ones are cueing you to eat.

Execute changes:
  ▷ Keep an eating diary and notice the patterns.
  ▷ Save this diary and use it for a reference in chapter 10.

PAUSE FOR WISDOM
*A crust eaten in peace is better than a
banquet partaken in anxiety.*
AESOP

10

THE POWER OF FOOD THOUGHTS

Take a minute and recall the opening story of this book about two friends talking at a coffee shop. One friend spotted a pastry in a glass case that looked delicious. As she sat and talked, all she could think about was the pastry and how good it would taste with her coffee. Eventually, she went to the counter and purchased the pastry.

This chapter addresses the role that thoughts play in our eating. How much does thinking about food influence our decisions to eat? Did it matter that the woman in the coffee shop continued to think about the pastry? Did her thoughts have anything to do with her behavior?

Recently I bought a bag of chocolates—which is okay to do. You can eat a piece of chocolate and not be a bad or weak-willed person!

My bag contained bite-sized pieces of dark chocolate with messages printed in the inside wrappers of each piece. So when you unwrap a piece, a message awaits you.

As I opened the wrapper of my piece of chocolate, I was curious about what wisdom would be imparted to me while I indulged in the delight. Written on the foil was "Don't think about it too much!"

I had to laugh because there was wisdom and folly in that shiny gold aluminum foil. Thinking about how good that chocolate was going to taste would influence my eating. So should I follow the advice of the chocolate and not think about it too much?

The Power of Our Thoughts

According to researcher Brian Wansink, PhD, in *Mindless Eating*,[1] just *thinking* that a meal will taste good makes you eat more. The more I thought about how tasty that chocolate was going to be, the more chocolates I would probably eat.

Apparently our minds are powerful when it comes to eating. The more premeditated the thought of an oncoming tasty treat, the more we are ready to receive. The more I look at the chocolate and think about how tasty it will be, the more likely I will be to eat it and additional pieces.

This is one of the reasons so many people struggle with eating. They are constantly anticipating a meal or thinking about what they will eat next. When they do this, they are setting themselves up to overeat.

So what would happen if I gave no thought to eating? What if I grabbed the chocolate and ate it without thinking at all? Would that be better than anticipating the melting delight in my mouth?

Apparently not! Giving no thought to what I am eating is also a problem. If I don't think at all about popping the chocolates into my mouth, I could end up eating a bunch of them because I'm eating unconsciously. So somewhere between thinking too much about the chocolate and not thinking at all, there is a balance. Like the message from the chocolate says, "Don't think about it *too much!*"

Our thoughts can and do trigger eating. And a thought can bring on an emotional state that leads to eating as well. It works like this:

We hold on to certain beliefs and assumptions about food that we have developed through our lives. Those beliefs result in automatic thoughts that come into our minds. Those thoughts influence how we feel (our emotions). Feelings influence how we behave. Then our behavior affects our perceptions. Our perceptions influence our thoughts. This loop continues to repeat.

The mind is powerful in how it influences feelings, behavior, and perceptions. It is in our thoughts that most eating battles are fought. Yet, our thoughts don't have to be constantly warring against us.

An old proverb says, "How you think in your heart is how you will be." In the proverb, "heart" is a reference to the mind. Thoughts influence our behavior. In particular, positive thoughts regarding food and eating can bring about a healthier view of both. Instead of hating our bodies because of how much we eat or seeing food as the enemy, we can develop a positive view of eating. We can move away from thinking of food negatively and choose new thoughts that will affect our emotions and behavior positively.

This is one reason the Bible talks so specifically about the power of the mind. Scriptures instruct us to think on things that are true, noble, reputable, authentic, compelling, and gracious. When we do this, the promise is that God makes everything work together and brings peace. Most of us could use a little more peace in our lives, especially when it comes to food thoughts.

Reflect on Your Thoughts

One of the problems we face in looking at our thoughts is that we are so distracted. We don't attend to our thoughts when eating. We allow distraction to take our minds in multiple directions. It seems that the last thing we think about is the food we are eating. Instead we are thinking about paying the babysitter, picking up the dry cleaning, and making it to the PTA meeting on time.

Because we have trouble focusing on the food we eat when we eat

A Maid-to-Order Exercise Program

Harvard researchers studied a group of female hotel room attendants. The researchers told part of the study group that the exercise they were getting from doing their jobs met or exceeded the recommended amount established by the government. These women believed that by doing their jobs, they were getting the exercise they needed to be healthy. The other group was not given this message. How did this message affect the behavior of the women?

Eighty percent of those who were told that their work met the guidelines for daily exercise reported exercising regularly, lost weight, and lowered their blood pressure and BMI. The positive mindset these workers developed from what they were told changed their bodies and behavior![2]

it, let's return to the quick exercise I mentioned in chapter 3 in which we practiced listening to our bodies for signs of hunger. Only this time, pay more attention to the thoughts that come into your mind when you eat. Aim at ridding yourself of distracting thoughts when eating. Concentrate on the act of eating. When you do this, observe your thoughts.

Choose a piece of fruit to eat. Focus only on that fruit. Look at it. Pick it up. Notice the texture, the color, and the smell and then take a bite. Now focus your mind. Close your eyes. Where are your thoughts? If they are wandering to your to-do list, bring them back to the task: eating a piece of fruit. Think only about the fruit—the taste, smell, and texture.

Did you notice how easily your mind wanders off to all kinds of things on your to-do list or to the details of your day? This is because we are so used to multitasking that we rarely concentrate on one thing at a time. Bring your attention full center to eating the fruit. Think about the luscious taste of the fruit and enjoy every bite. Chew it slowly. Enjoy the taste. This is eating with intention. It requires focusing your thoughts on the activity of eating.

Focusing on the food being eaten is one reason people in other cultures enjoy eating. They have learned to enjoy the moment and concentrate on the task at hand.

You may be thinking, *Big deal, what can this do for me?* Actually, it can do a lot. You are learning how to focus your attention and monitor your thoughts. Observe what specific thoughts go through your mind, and you may discover something. Perhaps your thoughts are critical and negative when you eat. *I can't have this. This is bad for me. I don't deserve to enjoy this.*

Thoughts to Watch Out For

Watch for these thoughts:

All or nothing. This type of thinking relates to dieting. With all-or-nothing thoughts, we judge ourselves as either perfect or a total failure. There is no in-between. Examples:

- ▶ *I can't eat foods with any fat in them.*
- ▶ *Eating dessert is bad for me.*
- ▶ *I ate a candy bar. I blew my diet completely.*
- ▶ *I ate too much for lunch, so I might as well eat whatever I want the rest of the day.*
- ▶ *I'm a failure. I ate a second piece of pizza last night.*

Catastrophic. You perceive one behavior as bigger than it is. Examples of catastrophic food thoughts:

- ▶ *My weight didn't even drop a pound this week. It doesn't matter what I eat.*

- *I sneaked two cookies, so I must be a binge eater.*
- *I ate an appetizer and a dessert, so I must be an overeater.*
- *I ate a candy bar and two cookies, so I'm going to gain weight.*

Pessimistic. You see the glass half empty rather than half full. Your thoughts are so negative about food and eating that they lead you to feel defeated. Examples of pessimistic thoughts:

- *The food in that restaurant was so greasy and terrible that I will probably get sick.*
- *I will never be able to control my craving for ice cream.*
- *I can't eat well when I eat out. It's too difficult.*
- *My family hates me when I cook healthful food like whole-wheat pasta.*

Self-fulfilling. You think you already know the outcome and believe it will be the same each time. This type of thinking about eating and food leads to discouragement. Examples of self-fulfilling thoughts:

- *I can't help myself. When I am stressed, I have to eat.*
- *I can't stop eating even when I am full.*
- *If I have potato chips, I have to eat the entire bag.*
- *When we go on our cruise, my eating will be out of control.*
- *If you ate my mother's cooking, you would be overweight, too.*

"Should." These thoughts require you to operate by rigid rules that usually set you up for a fall. They bring on regret and guilt. Examples:

- *I should eat only unprocessed food; if I don't, I will get sick.*
- *I should never eat sugar or I will gain weight.*

- *I should always choose the healthy dessert or I am a bad person.*
- *I should stop eating dessert.*

Blaming others. You fail to take responsibility for your actions and blame others. Assigning blame for your eating to other people results in a loss of personal responsibility. It assumes that you have no control over what you put in your mouth. Examples of blaming thoughts:

- *If it wasn't for my husband, I could lose weight.*
- *My mother taught me how to eat wrong, so I'm doomed.*
- *I have to eat when other people make me angry.*
- *If it wasn't for all the TV commercials, I could do better with snacking.*
- *If people at the office didn't bring in snacks, I could lose weight.*

Overgeneralizing. You think because something has happened before that it will happen again or recur frequently. Examples:

- *I overate last night; I'll never get control of my eating.*
- *My struggle with eating will be lifelong because my mother has a weight problem.*
- *When people upset me, I have to eat in order to calm down.*
- *When I eat dessert, I will overeat for the rest of the day.*
- *Because I am an emotional eater, I will be one for the rest of my life.*

Treat Unwanted Thoughts Like Computer Spam

When we are attuned to the moment, we are able to notice the thoughts that surface. I like to compare thoughts coming into my head with e-mail showing up in my electronic mailbox. On my computer, a lot of spam comes to my mailbox, but I only read the mail I choose. Thoughts are similar. Many go through our minds, but we decide which ones to click on.

Thoughts come and go influenced by our present, past, and future. We may have been told that we don't deserve things or should feel guilty if we eat a particular food. Maybe you were called fat or teased about your weight and have decided you are "bad" if you eat certain foods or weigh a particular amount. These experiences influence your thoughts about eating.

Or you may think that eating a certain food or allowing yourself a treat is bad because it will make you fat or gain weight. You might even think you don't deserve to feel pleasure. So your thoughts are constantly fixed on depriving yourself.

Rolinda struggled with thoughts about the future because of a family history of weight problems. She was convinced that eating desserts or any sweets would cause her weight to balloon up like her sisters. So every time she was presented with a dessert, her thoughts went like this: *I can't eat this or I will become fat like my sisters. Desserts are bad and will put weight on me.*

The truth is that desserts in moderation aren't bad. And that is the problem with our thinking. We don't consider moderation when it comes to eating. One dessert isn't going to make you gain a pound unless it contains more than 3,500 calories or puts you way over your calorie allotment for that day. When you stay within a healthy calorie count, a modest portion of dessert is fine. We don't have to be victims of our pasts or of fears about the future. Every moment is a new one. You can begin today to enjoy your food without clicking on the past or the future. However, this requires focus on your part and an understanding of the role that thoughts play in your behavior.

Identify the Belief and Thought

It is important to identify your thoughts about food and eating. Food is to be enjoyed and eating should be pleasurable. Allow your mind to agree with this point of view. If you continue to think of food as your enemy, you will struggle. Like the women who believed they were meeting their exercise goals while doing their jobs, believe that eating is a natural and good experience. Here is how you do this:

1. Identify any negative thoughts about food, such as, *Food is my enemy.*
2. Identify the thought you would like to think (something you know to be true), such as, *Food is designed for my health and enjoyment.*
3. Observe the times you have the negative thought, such as, *Every time I eat a dessert, I have the thought about food as my enemy.*
4. Don't click on that thought. Let it go and think a new thought, one that aligns with your positive belief about food and eating, such as, *Dessert is not my enemy. I can have it if I eat it in moderation. I can indulge as long as it doesn't increase my calories so much that I gain weight.*

To change your thoughts, examine your beliefs. Beliefs are those assumptions you hold about the world that shape your thoughts. If you believe deprivation is the key to curbing your eating, you will diet and struggle most of your life. If, however, you believe that food is acceptable, nourishing, and pleasurable, your behavior will follow this thought. Then you can eat without your thoughts triggering negative emotions.

If we really want to see the power of thoughts on behavior, let's revisit the biblical story of Eve in the Garden of Eden. Eve was tempted by a thought given to her by the serpent. When the serpent asked Eve to explain the directive God gave about eating the fruit, she told him, "We may eat fruit from the trees in the garden, but God did say, 'You must not eat fruit from the tree that is in the middle of the garden, and you must not touch it, or you will die.'" The serpent replies with a new thought, "You will not surely die" (3 Genesis NIV). Based on this new thought, Eve changed her belief. She agreed with a lie and the rest is history!

If you believe that eating must be a struggle or is in some way negative, your thoughts will be influenced by this belief. Your thoughts will then prompt negative feelings, behavior, or perceptions about food and eating. The key is to examine your beliefs that lead to your automatic thoughts. Identify one negative belief that has caused you problems. Here are some common negative beliefs regarding food and eating:

- *Food is my enemy.*
- *I must deprive myself of anything I enjoy.*
- *I can't eat or I will gain weight.*
- *I don't deserve to eat enjoyable foods.*
- *I can't allow myself to feel pleasure.*
- *I am a bad person for eating _____.*
- *Some foods are good, others are bad.*
- *Losing weight will make me happy and stop the pain.*
- *If I allow myself to eat, I'll never stop.*

Have you ever wondered why we have so many negative thoughts and not more positive ones when it comes to food and the way we feel about ourselves? One reason is that negative thoughts easily become reinforced in our minds. If we have insecurities, tend to compare ourselves to others, or operate with hurts and wounds, it is easy to think negatively. Our minds are receptive to negativity or false beliefs.

Too often we see ourselves in a bad light when it comes to eating.

We tend to think of eating as giving in to temptation, an addiction, or something out of our control. Our minds can be blinded, corrupted, debased, or hardened. This is why you should renew your thoughts daily, because they are so easily deceived by lies and negative words we encounter.

Replace your negative thoughts with more positive ones:

- *Overeating at a buffet does not make me a loser.*
- *I don't have to throw in the towel just because I snacked on pizza and wings.*
- *I don't have to beat myself up with thoughts of failure and deprivation so common to food and eating problems.*

Work on identifying your unhelpful food thoughts using the four steps outlined above. Over time, you can recognize negative food thoughts and change them to align with the belief that eating is pleasurable and enjoyable.

What is important is that you observe your thoughts and stop focusing on how bad you are or how necessary it is to deprive yourself of certain foods. Instead, remember to think about negative food thoughts as you would think about computer spam. If your thoughts are not helpful or are not in sync with your beliefs, don't "click" on them. Click on more positive thoughts that align with the belief that eating should be enjoyed.

How We Develop a Negative Relationship with Food

It is easy to develop negative thoughts about food in our culture. The messages we receive from other people, our experiences, our caretakers, and the media influence our thoughts if we don't regularly renew our mind with truth.

When we are babies, food is just food. Eating is a normal and natural part of the day. We are hungry and we are fed. We don't think too much about eating. Our main goal is to be fed and satisfied.

As we grow and develop, food takes on more complex meanings based on our experiences with caregivers and the context in which food is given. I worked with a woman whose mother was regularly depressed. Because of untreated debilitating depression, the mother rarely cooked. Instead, she opened cans of prepared food and served them at the table for meals. She would open a can of green beans, put a spoon in it, and serve it to the family. She did this with a variety of foods for most meals.

The children in this family developed negative associations with food. Because of the mother's depressed state, mealtimes were tense and unpleasant. The food, coming straight from the can, didn't taste good and was associated with depression. When the children thought about food, there was no joy and certainly no pleasure associated with mealtimes. Consequently, these kids developed eating problems. This is an extreme example, but it shows the influence of both caregivers and the context in which food is eaten.

Caretakers can also make remarks about food that influence your view of eating and the body. A mother who is constantly dieting in front of her teens teaches them that there is ongoing tension with food. On the positive side, caretakers can teach children a healthy way to think about food. Eating at a meal can be based on hunger cues and can be enjoyable with good conversation.

The larger culture also plays a role in shaping our food thoughts. With the incredible emphasis on thinness and beauty, we are over-focused on reaching unrealistic weight goals. We often believe that certain foods make us fat and that we should deprive ourselves for the sake of our body to meet cultural prescriptions of thinness. Our belief that we can always be thinner and improved leads us into unhealthy thinking about food. Food becomes the substance we want to control because we can't meet the unrealistic expectations presented to us.

We begin to believe that any type of eating puts on weight and that we have to constantly deny ourselves in order to be good enough. Consequently, we have record rates of people with body dissatisfaction, eating disorders, and obesity.

We war against our thoughts to be thinner and better. And while the battle appears to be based in obsessive thoughts about weight and dieting, the real struggle often involves underlying issues around identity and relationships. Until we recognize that our obsessive food thoughts represent deeper problems, we will continue to obsess and use food in unhealthy ways.

Add to our inner struggles the distorted and confusing messages of media, and it is easy to see how a negative relationship with food develops.

Be Compassionate with Yourself

When it comes to eating, many of us find an inner critic who is always commenting and chiding us about what we eat. If that is you, it's time to silence the critic. Replace the critic with words of compassion and understanding. Let's stop judging ourselves harshly and understand the significant role that thoughts play in our sense of well-being.

To better understand the role that the inner critic plays in our lives, we can look at someone who struggles with bulimia. The inner critic of a bulimic person is loud and active.[3] According to the *International Journal of Eating Disorders*, bulimics tend to have thoughts about shame and feeling defective, about failure, and about lacking self-control. As the inner critic speaks loudly, food is used to silence those critical thoughts that cause distressing emotional feelings.

A person with bulimia needs to think differently about eating. She needs to know that unbridled eating leads to obesity and health problems, and obsession leads to eating disorders. In the middle of those two extremes is a view that sees food as necessary and helpful to our bodies. Food sustains our health and is a part of our daily routine.

When a bulimic begins to reexamine her beliefs and thoughts about food and eating and begins to recognize the need to silence the inner critic, she is on the road to recovery. And while most of us may not have the thought distortions of a bulimic, we still allow the inner critic to speak loudly. We too have to learn to silence that voice and listen to a kinder, more compassionate voice.

So examine your beliefs about your body and eating. Are they unrealistic, too harsh, perfectionist, self-defeating, or distorted? Do you think thoughts like, *I ate a candy bar today, so I blew it. I may as well eat whatever I want for the rest of this day?*

If so, you need more compassion when it comes to taking care of yourself. Better to think, *Okay, I had a candy bar. One will not make me gain a pound. It wasn't 3,500 calories! I'm okay.* Seize the moment to be kind to yourself.

Why Resistance Isn't the Answer

So many of our thoughts about eating involve resisting. *Resist that chocolate dessert. Don't give in to that mile-high plate of nachos. Resist!* But when it comes to eating, resistance isn't always the best path.

Resistance is exhausting. One of the reasons we like diets is because we grow tired of thinking about food and just want someone to tell us what to do. Diets are enticing because they prescribe how we are to eat. We don't have to make choices. We don't have to think. Someone else is directing our food choices.

The problem is that over time we resist being told what to do and want to take back control. In the long term, we don't do well with other people directing what goes into our mouths. So the strategy to restrain our eating through dieting doesn't usually work when it comes to thinking about food. Remember, the more we try not to think about the food, the more we will think about it. A University of Hertfordshire study[4] demonstrated that men and women who try to resist thoughts about eating chocolate, eat more chocolate.

Recall that food thoughts come and go during our everyday lives. A food thought is not a problem unless you focus on it and begin to visualize that mouthwatering snack you think you must have. The more you think about a food and decide you *can't* have it, the more you want it.

So allow thoughts about food to flow through your mind. Then be curious about your thoughts instead of fighting them. Ask why you are having that thought. Are you trying to distract yourself from an emotion or to extend a happy feeling? Are you feeling so sorry for yourself or so angry that you want to eat pizza? Be curious about what is motivating the thought of food at any given moment.

If hunger is your motivation, go ahead and eat, but choose your foods and portion size with conscious thought. Otherwise, observe the thought and see what it triggers in you. Try not to judge your thoughts or feelings related to food. Allow them to surface. Someone once said, "Whatever you resist, will persist." Don't resist.

In a classic study regarding thought suppression published in the *Journal of Personality and Social Psychology*,[5] researchers from collaborating universities showed subjects a movie about white bears. Subjects were then divided into two groups. One group was told not to think about the white bears and the other group was given no such instruction. The group told to suppress the thought of white bears actually thought more about them than the other group.

So when you have the urge to eat and can only think about the craving, try to allow that thought instead of suppressing it. Don't fight it. Soon the thought will pass if you let it be. Fighting the craving usually ends up in giving it more time and attention than necessary. That attention can lead you to eat.

If the urge returns later, do the same. Allow the thought without trying to resist it. Eventually it will pass. However, it is important to know that when you allow an urge to exist, it sometimes grows stronger. But if you do nothing, it will eventually go away. If you give in, it will increase in intensity again.

This doesn't mean you are doomed if you give in to an eating urge. Rather, it means that when you do give in, the urge will feel strong the next time. If you allow the thought to come and go and do nothing with it, eventually it won't be reinforced and will pass.

When you have the urge to eat and allow yourself to accept whatever thought or feeling emerges, describe what you noticed. What was the thought? Are you judging yourself or mistaking opinion for fact? Stick with the facts (for example, *Is this what I think or know to be true?*) Try to balance your thoughts and feelings so that neither takes over.

What you are doing is experiencing the urge in a new way—not fighting it or trying desperately to resist, but allowing it, accepting it without judgment, and letting it pass. Urges are like waves. They come and go, crest and subside. They begin small and build in size but eventually break up like a wave on the shore. Your job is to ride the wave, not fight it. Focus on the urge. Be curious about it, not anxious.

Sometimes it helps to categorize thoughts. Did you have a worrisome thought, a happy thought, an angry thought? Once you become aware of the thought and feeling, write it down. Your objective is to understand which thoughts or feelings trigger you to eat. If you are reacting to a specific thought or feeling, you can practice doing something other than eating at that moment. Or you can change the thought to one that aligns with your beliefs. Allow yourself to experience the thought but don't act on it in the old way (more on this in chapter 13).

Reconsider Your Reactions

Remember your eating diary from chapter 9, where you tracked the feeling that led you to eat? Now, we want to add to that diary the *thought* that might trigger the emotion or the eating behavior. For example:

SITUATION	WHAT DO I THINK?	WHAT DO I FEEL?	DID I EMOTIONALLY EAT?
My husband yelled at me.	*He thinks I am stupid.*	Hurt	Yes
My boss criticized me.	*He thinks he is better than I am.*	Anger	Yes
Conflict with a friend.	*She won't speak to me again.*	Rejection	Yes

Notice that all three of these thought examples involve judgments—judgments based on your opinion. Negative opinions usually lead us to feel bad and trigger eating.

If we revisit the same situations and try to be more descriptive in our thoughts, we may have different results. For example, when my husband yells at me, I could think, *He's very upset. I wonder what is wrong.* This thought is nonjudgmental. It is a description of what is seen rather than an opinion of what might be happening. And if you are like me, I can't read minds!

Judgments or opinions serve to work us up emotionally, and our emotions take over. We then lose our ability to think clearly and respond differently. So try to stay with a description of what happened and then identify your feeling.

Using the second example, "My boss criticized me," one could think, *Maybe there is a reason for this,* or *I don't really understand why he did this since I don't know what I did wrong.* These thoughts are not judgment based or opinion based. They are thoughts that attempt to clarify a behavior.

The third example, a conflict with a friend, reveals a fear of possible rejection. This may be based on past experience, but rather than judging and assuming the negative, wait and see what happens.

If she does surprise you and speaks to you, you've avoided feeling rejected. And if she does avoid you and you feel rejected, remember that there are ways other than eating to handle rejection.

Notice Your Patterns

After keeping this type of eating diary for a few weeks, you will begin to see patterns in not only your feelings but in the thoughts that trigger your emotions. Awareness increases your understanding of which thoughts and emotions trigger unintentional eating. Then you can learn to anticipate, allow, and deal better with these thoughts and emotions. And remember, food does not have to be your coping mechanism.

Wendy learned how to reconsider her reactions. When her husband argued with her recently, her initial thought was, *My husband is a jerk*, which was a judgmental thought. She changed her thought to one that was nonjudgmental and more descriptive: *My husband argued with me and it makes me uncomfortable because he usually won't bend his opinion. I wonder if this time could be different and we could actually have a reasonable conversation about our differences.*

Wendy still felt uncomfortable with the conflict but rather than grabbing a candy bar to calm down, she could be more assertive and confront her husband's argumentative behavior. She had to make a decision. Would she act on the discomfort by eating or confront her husband about his behavior? Before she even got to the decision part, however, she decided to handle her thoughts differently. She described what she saw and withheld judgment until she could have a clarifying conversation.

Now which is easier? Eating the candy bar or confronting a spouse? Most people would choose the candy bar, but to break the pattern of unintentional eating, choose to be assertive. (We'll cover this in more depth in chapter 14.)

Your thoughts are important: be curious about your food thoughts.

When you identify negative thoughts, you may feel anxious at first. Any time we become more aware of our behavior, it can initially make us more anxious. Over time, you will become more comfortable with your thoughts, knowing you can allow them or change them and react less impulsively. You can learn to withhold judgments and behave differently.

Understanding your thought life makes you accountable for the decision whether to hang on to your negative thoughts or to do something about them. *Press pause* and examine your thoughts.

THE PRESS PAUSE PRINCIPLE

Plan to examine your eating and food thoughts.

Attend to your food thoughts and determine if they are negative, opinion based, or judgmental.

Understand that food thoughts are powerful precursors to the way we feel and act. Trying to suppress food thoughts usually leads to thinking about them even more and results in more eating.

Strategize: identify your food thoughts by tracking them in an eating diary. Notice any patterns or regularly occurring thoughts that lead to eating.

Execute changes:

▷ Change your belief about eating in order to develop a more positive relationship with food and eating.

▷ Allow your food thoughts to come and go. Don't judge them. Ride them out and be curious about them. Eventually they will subside. They are only thoughts. Silence the inner critic and be more compassionate to yourself.

PAUSE FOR WISDOM

For many, negative thinking is a habit, which over time, becomes an addiction. . . . A lot of people suffer from this disease because negative thinking is addictive to each of the Big Three—the mind, the body, and the emotions. If one doesn't get you, the others are waiting in the wings.

PETER McWILLIAMS

11

SPIRITUAL HUNGER REQUIRES SPIRITUAL FOOD

Have you ever had a desire for a certain food and nothing but that food would satisfy you? Perhaps all you can think about is having a hot fudge sundae. You try not to think about it, but thoughts of that sundae continue to be in your brain. No matter what you do, nothing helps. You have to have the hot fudge sundae and will go to great lengths to get it.

What you are experiencing is a food craving. We tend to have them more often when we restrict our eating or our eating becomes boring and monotonous. This is one reason why sticking to a restrictive diet rarely works. Researchers at the Monell Chemical Senses Center and the University of Pennsylvania School of Medicine[1] found that the more bored we become with the foods we allow, the more we crave foods we really like. Food cravings aren't just our imaginations. They are linked to the brain and hormones. And without being aware of it, we can crave foods associated with food memories. When it comes to the brain, food cravings activate the same parts of the brain as drug cravings do. These areas of the brain involve memory, rewards, and emotions.

It works like this. We have a craving for a food based on a food memory. For example, I may crave berry pies because I have a pleasant food memory associated with them. And that craving will be satisfied by only that food because I have satisfied it with that food in the past. We have memories of a particular food meeting a need. And we are creatures of habit who tend to go back to things that involve reward or pleasant memories.

We have already learned that food and emotions can be paired to meet emotional needs. This chapter explores how food and spiritual cravings can also be paired.

Trying to Fill a Void

Are there times when we eat due to an emptiness that has nothing to do with food?

Is there something deep inside us that only a robust spiritual life can fill? Do we crave meaning and purpose that can't be attained by things we buy or accomplish? Do we sense there is more to life than what we can see? If you answered yes to any of these questions, you are beginning to recognize spiritual cravings.

Spiritual cravings involve the intangible: those things we long for in order to live a meaningful and purposeful life. Like food cravings, only specific things will satisfy. So when we try to satisfy spiritual cravings with solutions unrelated to spiritual food, we are left empty and dissatisfied.

There is something in all of us that craves a spiritual connection. The problem is we don't always recognize this craving and we often mistake it for other things. The following conversation with Fran gives us a hint as to how spiritual cravings can be mistaken for food.

Fran craved fresh chocolate chip cookies like her mother used to make. Eating them made her feel calm and peaceful. When she thought about her family, she recalled how strong her parents were in their faith, and that she craved that spiritual strength perhaps more than she craved the cookies.

Fran: Right now I have the craving for chocolate chip cookies—fresh out of the oven, creamy, warm, and chewy chocolate chip cookies like the ones my mom used to bake.

Dr. Linda: What about those cookies is so inviting?

Fran: They are rich, warm, and melt in my mouth. And they remind me of home.

Dr. Linda: When you have those warm, rich, melt-in-your-mouth cookies, what are you feeling?

Fran: Calm and peaceful. I think about the family in which I was raised. We had our problems but most of the time, we got along and had peace in our home. My parents were very strong in their faith and no matter what happened, they turned to God for help. Because of their faith, I always believed things would work out. I guess I felt secure.

Dr. Linda: So your desire is not only for the cookies but to feel that peace and calm again, to be loved and feel secure?

Fran: I've never thought about it like that. I guess so. But don't I just want the cookies?

Dr. Linda: You tell me. What is your wish for your life right now?

Fran: I would really like to feel that peace I felt when I was with my mom baking cookies. Now, there is so much chaos in my home. We don't cope very well with problems and we don't include God in anything. We don't acknowledge that God even exists but I believe he does. I don't like feeling like this so I guess the cookies do give me the feelings I want—at least for the moment. That sounds so weird to even say!

Dr. Linda: Do you think peace and calm are possible in your life today?

Fran: No, not really.

Dr. Linda: What would happen if you were honest about desiring that peace and calm? Would that be okay?

Fran: It would be wonderful but it's unrealistic given my current situation. I don't want to wish for something that I can't have. I'll only be disappointed. And I'd rather not feel that at all.

Dr. Linda: So you would rather give up on the wish for peace and calm and go for the cookies?

Fran: Not when you put it that way.

Dr. Linda: Are you afraid to want something you don't think you can have, or afraid to admit to the desire for peace and calm in your home? Desiring this is a worthy and attainable goal. Together, there are steps we can take to cultivate peace and calm in your family if you admit to your longing and stop using the cookies as a substitute.

Fran: I would like that. I've always wondered if my cravings were bigger than the food, but honestly, I didn't want to think about that too much. As an adult, I've avoided thinking about my spiritual life even though it was important to me as a child. I don't want to admit to many things because I know it will mean changes for me.

Dr. Linda: You are probably right. Cookies are much easier!

Fran expressed a food craving that was more than a biological urge. She was spiritually hungry and didn't recognize it. Food became her channel to fill a spiritual emptiness. But cookies can't do the job, no matter how tasty they are. They are only a temporary fix for a deeper longing.

Intuitively Fran knew that eating cookies wasn't an answer to the void she felt in her life. When Fran pressed *pause* and was honest about her inner life, she admitted to an unmet spiritual need. She longed for the peace she once felt in her home. Cookies were only a memory that unlocked a bigger need. Fran once lived in a home in which people of faith had a positive impact on her life. Religion was not some vain repetition or empty ritual performed at a church or temple. Authentic faith was lived out in Fran's family life and she witnessed the transformation it made in the people she loved. Her family was far from perfect but the spiritual climate in her home was one of peace.

Fran never made her parents' faith her own. When she married, she didn't think spirituality was important to creating a successful life. She soon realized there was something missing, something she couldn't put her finger on but sensed was lacking. With a little prob-ing, Fran was able to articulate the void she felt and decided to ex-plore her spiritual roots.

Fran had to stop pretending that the void she felt could be ig-nored or filled with cookies. She did have cravings, but cookies were only a cover-up for deeper wishes.

Fran wasn't sure that her spiritual cravings could be satisfied at this time. She was wrong. Fulfilling this need was not dependent on circumstances or the actions of her husband. She could embrace her faith and find what she longed for—peace and contentment despite her circumstances. And she could stop using food in a way she never intended.

Behind many of our food desires is a longing for something we've yet to identify. It takes a moment, a pause, to think about what that could be. If you are searching for meaning, purpose, love, validation, acceptance, security, or belonging, you may be spiritually hungry. This is a type of hunger that will never be met through warm and chewy chocolate chip cookies!

Fran was looking for something beyond herself that could give her a sense of peace and security. In a sermon published in *The Weight of Glory*, C. S. Lewis described this type of desire as "the scent of a flower we have not found, the echo of a tune we have not heard, news from a country we have never visited." Lewis was referring to a desire for completion that cannot be met through food or any other natural means.

Spiritual hunger involves a craving for something beyond food or any other pleasure. It is that sense that our human bodies were meant for something more than we can summon them to do. We feel a pull to something we cannot see but is bigger than we are. Simply put, this is our desire for a rich spiritual life.

Our desire for God is something we were created to feel. It is not a desire that must be stopped or transcended, but embraced because it ultimately brings satisfaction to our lives. However, we can seek to fulfill this desire in ways that will never bring true satisfaction or rest. This happens when we try to complete ourselves apart from God, when we fall for the modern-day delusion that we are self-sufficient.

But God desires us, and that is the beauty of the desire. We are easily found by him. He has been waiting for us and desires us to make our home with him. When we agree to this residence, he begins to fill us up with purpose, meaning, love, acceptance, belonging, security, and other abundant spiritual food.

This craving we have for meaning and purpose can be satisfied by answering the call God has on our lives. Apologist Os Guinness defines calling as "the truth that God calls us to himself so decisively that everything we are, everything we do, and everything we have is invested with such a special devotion and dynamism lived out as a response to his summon and service." We can't complete this calling until we engage with the One who calls us. It is through our intimate relationship with God that we fulfill our reason for existence. When craving meets Creator, fulfillment happens.

When we are intimate with God, we realize that he knows us individually and uniquely. He has arranged our destiny but wants to partner with us for the journey. With God, we are continuously becoming who he intended us to be. And the more we can get ourselves out of the way and let God do his magnificent work in us, the better the results.

When we become one of God's followers, we understand an even deeper truth. This world isn't the final stop in our journey through life. There is more beyond this present day. And there is an excitement in our spirits for that day of completion. We long for this day when we are transformed from glory to glory.

Augustine said, "You [God] have made us for yourself, and our hearts are restless until they find their rest in you." Without God, a spiritual life, we are restless and incomplete because we were made for intimacy with him. He draws us to him and waits to complete us. However, it is up to us to decide if we will accept this incredible invitation. He waits with spiritual food, but we must go to his banqueting table.

Babette's Feast

One of my favorite movies is an endearing foreign film entitled *Babette's Feast*, directed by Gabriel Axel. The movie takes place in a small coastal Danish town where twin sisters live a pious life as daughters of a Lutheran minister who founded a religious sect.

The sisters, Martina and Philippa, relinquished their chances for romance and adventure in their youths to follow their father's religion. Their lives are austere, with little enjoyment. Enjoying food was frowned upon. Cooking was plain and the money saved from preparing meager meals was given to the poor.

Babette, a political refugee from France, arrives in the town and begs the sisters to allow her to live with them and be their housekeeper. Unbeknownst to the sisters, Babette is an exquisite chef from Paris.

The sisters' father dies and they decide to throw a feast in order to honor and commemorate his life. Times have been tough, leading to tension in the small congregation.

(continued)

Babette, who has won the lottery, decides to use all of her money to honor the memory of this man by preparing an elaborate feast for the members of his tiny church. Babette convinces the sisters to allow her to take charge of the celebration. The sisters concede to her request.

The feast Babette prepares is one that church members will never forget. However, they come to the meal determined not to enjoy it, since part of their religious lifestyle is to renounce the pleasures of this world. As Babette unleashes her cooking talents on those who are reluctant to receive, the group loosens up and receives this tremendous gift. The feast is elaborate and divine, and relationship healings and reconciliation are unexpected outcomes.

One of the multiple layers of meaning has to do with the sterile and pious lives the sisters live in response to a religion that requires no sensual enjoyment or celebration. Babette teaches them that living piously does not require renouncing all enjoyment or celebration. She offers all she has—the ability to create a sensual feast for all. It is through the preparation of food and the pleasure of eating that people can relax and enjoy the moment.

Babette's feast demonstrates that where there was once bitterness, gratitude can abound. Where fear and suspicion lived, trust can take over. Like the sisters, we are reminded of the true meaning of spirituality and the impact it has in our lives. The spiritual life brings completion to all that we were created to be.

Searching for Self

Our desire for God can be ignored. Spiritual cravings can be covered up. To fulfill our hunger, we can look to not only food but also other people. However, looking to others to satisfy spiritual hungers will bring only disappointment and despair.

Leslie always felt like she didn't belong. As an only child, her parents seemed distracted and too busy to be involved in her life. She spent many days alone in her bedroom wishing she had friends and a social life. In many ways, she was starved for attention.

Leslie desperately wanted companionship. When a classmate started paying attention to her, she noticed. Jake seemed like a nice guy who was everything she was not—outgoing, confident, and connected. Jake made her feel special.

The two began to date. Leslie could hardly believe her good fortune and felt as though Jake completed her. Whatever she lacked, he had. In Leslie's mind, the two of them were good together. He was the catalyst who brought her out of her shell, who could make her laugh and cared about her feelings. In turn, she helped Jake stay focused. Leslie decided she needed Jake in her life.

But Leslie's need began to grow and she soon felt like she couldn't function without Jake. When he didn't call, she became anxious. If he talked to other girls, she was jealous. The more she depended on him, the more desperate she became. All she could think about was how she needed Jake.

Leslie began to eat out of anxiety. She was afraid that her boyfriend was losing interest in her. Didn't he know how much she depended on him to make her smile and brighten her day? Didn't he realize that he was her lifeline? Without him, Leslie didn't want to exist. She turned to food for comfort and developed food cravings, cravings she felt she had to deny because she wasn't good enough to accept pleasure.

The needier she became, the more Jake distanced himself from the relationship. Because the emptiness Leslie felt was more than she could bear, eating became her solution to the void she felt. It was as if a part of her had been lost when Jake stopped calling.

When Leslie entered therapy, she was convinced that she needed this young man to complete who she was. Her longing for love, attention, and belonging was misdirected. No man could give her the confidence she lacked in terms of her identity. And restricting herself from the pleasure of food was not a solution that brought relief.

Like Leslie, we often look to others to give us what we think we are missing. That is a tall order for anyone and a recipe for an unhealthy relationship.

Our identity can only be found through a spiritual connection. When we realize that God wants to be the source of our confidence, we can relax and throw our dependence on him. He doesn't get tired of our neediness and distance as a result. In fact, he wants to meet our needs and give us a sense of self that can't be shaken by other people or circumstances. He encourages our dependence. Our confidence is in him, working in our lives for our good. Sometimes we think that being spiritual means giving up things and having a boring or austere life. Actually the opposite is true. A vibrant spiritual life brings joy and celebration as there is much more to gain than lose.

We lose anxiety, fear, and feelings of hopelessness. Life that was meaningless becomes purposeful. We are no longer driven because we recognize that we are called. The spiritual life is far from boring. It is an unfolding adventure filled with twists and turns.

It is possible to mistake spiritual hunger for food cravings. The longing that is in each of us to connect to something bigger than we are can leave us with a void if we don't fill it. But the void is spiritually based and must be filled with a vibrant spiritual life, not with food.

Press pause and reflect on your spiritual life. Do you have one? Have you ignored the spiritual part of who you are? Do you yearn for greater meaning and purpose in your life? Perhaps it is time to pursue a spiritual life that brings joy and meaning.

THE PRESS PAUSE PRINCIPLE

Plan in your heart to consider spiritual hunger.

Attend to feelings of restlessness, boredom, lack of purpose, and discontent.

Understand that spiritual hunger requires feeding with spiritual food.

Strategize how to develop a fulfilling spiritual life.

Execute changes:
  ▷ Accept and enjoy a rich spiritual life.

PAUSE FOR WISDOM
The meaning of our existence is not invented
by ourselves, but rather detected.
VIKTOR FRANKL, *MAN'S SEARCH FOR MEANING*

PART FOUR

STRATEGIZE

Now that we have learned to pause, to attend to the moment, to understand our thoughts, emotions, and spiritual lives, we can make changes that will create a positive and enjoyable relationship with food and eating. Each of us knows where we need to focus.

This section highlights more useful strategies that will help us eat with intention and feel positive about the role of eating in our lives. We will focus on three areas of change that are essential to developing a healthy relationship with food:

1. Refocus your view and renew your mind.
2. Regulate and tolerate your emotions.
3. Become more interpersonally effective.

The more we are able to do these three things, the less likely we will be to use food for hungers that are not physical.

12

TACKLE YOUR EMOTIONS

Let's look at the attitude of three people who struggle with their weight. Jim says, "I'll never get past using food to help me feel better. I'm a failure when it comes to getting control over food. I've tried many times to change but can't do it."

Jim is stuck and won't move forward because he is wallowing in his distress. He thinks like a victim and will stay miserable. He can question his plight and never move beyond the victim stage. Basically, he can keep asking, *Why me?* He has the choice to stay miserable and accept failure for what it is—failure.

Jane says, "I eat for all kinds of emotional reasons. I've been like this my whole life. I know I have a problem, but it's been too many years to change now."

Jane at least admits she has a problem. However, her response isn't much better than Jim's. She won't move beyond acceptance. She defines herself as an emotional eater, take it or leave it. Nonsense! Change is always possible. If you want to change, you can. It's your choice.

Emily says, "I know I emotionally eat, but I want to break the pattern. Isn't this a problem that can be solved? Other people do it."

Okay, now we have something to work with in terms of change. With this attitude, change is possible and emotional eating can be solved. But you have to want to do it.

When eating is the main response to emotions, we have to learn to respond other ways.

Eating lifts our mood and helps manage our emotions. One of the reasons we hesitate to give up emotional eating is because it works temporarily to fend off uncomfortable feelings or to celebrate positive ones. When you have something that works, it is not easy to let go of it.

Eating is easier than learning how to manage and tolerate emotions. It helps us avoid dealing with difficult emotions. An ice cream cone takes our mind off a bad day at work. A bag of chips can break feelings of boredom. Food distracts us. It gives us something other than our discomfort to focus on.

We've also seen how we express happy feelings through food. So the challenge is to not only manage and tolerate distressing feelings but to also express happiness and celebration in ways that don't always involve eating.

Why We Need to Face Our Feelings

Whatever our fears, we must put them in perspective. Feelings don't destroy us. No matter how deeply we hurt, how angry we become, or how long we grieve, it is not feelings that cause us to eat half of a pizza. It is the *avoidance* of uncomfortable feelings that brings trouble.

We want not only to become aware of what we feel, but also to allow those feelings to surface. When we do, it is important not to judge a feeling as right or wrong, good or bad. Just allow yourself to experience your feelings without putting food in your mouth.

To do so, you can't be afraid to feel. It is possible to learn to tolerate feelings.

When you allow feelings to surface, they eventually subside. And when feelings linger, you won't die, fall apart, or become bedridden once you learn to tolerate them. You may need help to learn to deal with them, but you will. In time, you can give up eating as a way to cope with uncomfortable emotions and use healthier ways to manage or tolerate all feelings. You have many tools available to you. Read on!

Begin with a Self-Reminder

To stop feasting on our emotions, begin with a simple strategy, backed by a study conducted at Case Western Reserve University in Cleveland, Ohio. In the study,[1] researchers induced a sad mood in two groups of people. When people felt sad, one group was told that even though they may think eating makes them feel better, science shows it doesn't. The other group wasn't told anything and ate more than the group that believed eating would not help them feel better.

Beliefs are powerful and affect how we behave. When we are emotionally distressed, we can remind ourselves that eating is not going to help us feel better. We won't feel better in the long run by downing an order of fries. According to the study, simply reminding ourselves of this truth may prevent us from eating.

So next time you reach for that third slice of pizza after a hard day at work, pause, and ask yourself, *Do I really want a third slice?* If your answer is, *Yes, it will make me feel better,* pause again. Tell yourself, *This will not improve my mood.* Then do something that will pick up your mood, such as listening to music, taking a walk, or playing with your pet. Over time, you will break the habit of emotional eating.

Self-reminders are a tool used to break the habit of emotional eating. In addition, a number of other skills will help you not turn to food when emotional, distressed, or happy.

Develop Emotional Rescues

Renee desperately wanted to stop eating in response to her emotions. We decided to tackle her problem by using healthy distractions, or what she called emotional rescues. Each time Renee was tempted to eat in an attempt to escape uncomfortable feelings, she chose from a list of emotional rescues and engaged in one of them instead of eating.

Renee made a list of twenty items she could use as distractions:

1. Walk around the block.
2. Talk to someone on e-mail, MySpace, or in a chat room.
3. Talk to someone on the phone.
4. Meet a friend at the local bookstore.
5. Take a nap.
6. Take a hot bath or shower.
7. Play music on a CD player.
8. Play music on an instrument.
9. Draw or paint.
10. Write a grocery list.
11. Write a letter to a friend.
12. Play cards.
13. Clean something.
14. Play a computer game.
15. Watch television (click off the commercials).
16. Pray.
17. Meditate on the goodness of God.
18. Play with the dog.
19. Count to ten and back several times.
20. Finish a chore.

The idea was to get Renee's mind off the food and on to something else that wouldn't cause her distress. Renee listed several emotional rescues. Each time she felt an uncomfortable emotion that typically led her to eat, she substituted an emotional rescue from the list. Here are a few of her examples:

Anger: Renee would listen to her iPod and sing along very loudly.

Worry: Renee would turn off the nightly news and watch a comedy or listen to a comic on a CD.

Sad: Renee would play something lively on the piano or read an up-beat psalm from her Bible.

Lonely: Renee logged on to Facebook and chatted with friends, e-mailed friends, or sent a text message.

Renee forced herself to choose an emotional rescue rather than eat. Over time, she broke the habit of pairing food with emotions.

You can do the same. Make a list of emotional rescues that would work to distract you from food. Post them on the refrigerator. List three to five that work well when the urge to emotionally eat hits. It helps to have emotional rescues that work in the car, at the office, at home, or wherever you struggle. If you have the urge to eat driving past the 7-Eleven because you just got cut off in traffic and are fuming, you can't distract yourself by taking a walk. You need a car strategy, such as listening to a book on tape or choosing a route that doesn't pass by the 7-Eleven. Develop your list and begin to use it.

Ways to Cope with Emotional Distress

Emotional rescues won't solve whatever triggered that emotion in the first place, but will help regulate your attention away from food. And they help break the pairing of food and feelings.

Use Social Support

When you are in the thick of stress or feel as if you are just reacting to your emotions, it may help to phone a friend or simply talk to someone nearby. Social support is helpful when trying to break the habit of eating mindlessly in response to emotions.

A friend can ask, "Are you really hungry right now or is something else going on?" Friends can be strong supports when you have the urge to eat without thinking. Give them permission to ask you *why* you want to eat. Asking this question is enough to slow down most people. With a pause, you can talk it out and decide not to eat at that moment. You can also identify the emotions and experience them without turning to food.

Social support can come from friends, family, or groups. As long as you aren't meeting people at the doughnut counter, you will find good support in those who agree to help you become more mindful.

Journal or Write in a Diary

If you can pause and process your feelings by writing, then journaling is for you. Reach for a pen instead of that chocolate bar next time you feel like mindlessly eating, and focus on how you feel and why you want to eat at that moment. Write instead of eat. Journaling is also a great way to record your progress and expand your awareness of self.

Get Some Exercise

Next time you walk mindlessly to the refrigerator, open the door, and stare at the inside contents, close the door and do a few jumping jacks. Exercise helps get your mind off of food. If you can make yourself exercise, the urge to eat will subside.

You may simply not enjoy exercising. That said, you can still do it. I don't enjoy swallowing vitamins every morning but I do so because I believe they are good for me. I don't enjoy weeding the garden but it will become overrun if I don't.

Exercise has many benefits, including de-stressing you. Next time you want to reach for the pint of ice cream, grab the dog's leash and take her for a walk. Not only will you avoid extra calories but you will be working them off. And walking can help you relax your body and tolerate stress.

Listen To or Play Music

When sitting at my computer becomes so boring I want to eat, I go to my piano and play. The distraction is great and it makes my parents proud to know that I actually use all those music lessons they paid for! Music has the potential to transport us, to move us, to relax us, to engage us away from food.

A friend of mine, Steve Siler, has a nonprofit organization called Music for the Soul. His mission is to provide life-changing healing through music and song. He believes that music is the language of the heart and mind, a universal language that speaks to all people. I couldn't agree more. Music soothes us and speaks to our souls and spirit. It is not only distracting from eating but can be healing as well.

Take a Bath or Long Steamy Shower, or Get a Massage

Any one of these options works for me! Baths and showers are such great substitutes for eating partly because the bathroom is not typically associated with food. In fact, I used to send my compulsive overeating clients to the bathroom when they had urges to eat. It was the one room in the house in which they did not have a history of eating and served as a cue to stop and think. A shower, bath, or massage is also relaxing and will slow you down so you can think about your behavior, relax your body, and practice tolerating distress.

Play an Electronic Game

While I am not a fan of long hours of screen time (video game playing and obesity are linked), you can jump on your computer or an electronic game device for a few minutes to distract yourself from the urge to eat.

As long as you don't sit there for hours and look up recipe sites, your mind will be distracted from thoughts of food. Again, be careful not to exchange one problem for another. Substituting the urge to eat for viewing pornography, engaging in racy chat, or spending long hours in front of a screen is not a desirable solution to mindless eating.

Clean or Do Chores

When I have been sitting a long time and get bored and want to eat, I clean. It is good exercise, needs to be done, and gets my mind off food. I highly recommend it! You feel productive and it burns calories.

Brush Your Teeth

An easy way to curb the urge to mindlessly eat is to brush your teeth. When we brush our teeth, it is a cue to stop eating. Brushing signals the end of eating, not the beginning. And afterward, drink a big glass of water to curb your impulse as well.

Engage in Relaxation and Prayer

Prayer and relaxation are great helps when it comes to pausing and thinking about what we do. King David, in the Old Testament of the

To Shop or Not to Shop?

Many people shop as a way to soothe themselves when upset. But is shopping really an advisable form of emotional rescue? Shopping may lead to debt or wasteful buying. If you can shop and stick to your budget or decide not to buy anything, this may work when you feel down or need to get out of the house and away from food. However, many shopping centers have tempting food smells, food courts, and coffee bars. So if you use shopping as a substitute for eating, make sure you aren't trading one bad habit for another. Shopping addiction can lead to debt and an overemphasis on materialism if you are not careful. And don't go food shopping when you feel emotionally distressed!

Bible, prayed for God to examine his heart and know his thoughts. Prayer can be a time of introspection, of asking God to reveal your true thoughts and hurts. If you can wait before God, good things will happen.

When we pray, we gain strength because we are partnering with God and asking him to be involved in our lives. Prayer also revives and refreshes us. We shift the burden or weight of our distress to God, who is more than willing to take it. Prayer is handing over the heavy load to God, leaving it with him and trusting him to work on our behalf and help us through difficulty. It is an underutilized resource.

Relaxation exercises such as breathing, muscle relaxation, and clearing the mind of stressful thoughts are another way to manage uncomfortable emotions. Take a quiet walk and relax your body and mind as you focus on nature and the blessings in your life. Sit quietly and focus on all the good things you have. Concentrate on relaxing your body, and thoughts of food will disappear. We have a hard time being still in American society but need to do it to refuel.

In addition to using these emotional rescues, it helps to have healthier food alternatives on hand for those times when you decide to give in to the urge to eat. Stock your refrigerator with sparkling water instead of soda, crisp vegetables and low-fat dips instead of chips, crunchy apples instead of butter-laden popcorn, and pieces of dark chocolate instead of chocolate cake.

There will be times when you choose to eat to cope. We all do it from time to time. Remember that your ultimate goal is not to use food for emotional comfort. So try the alternatives and practice pairing your emotions with other distractions in order to break the association with food.

Ways to Tolerate Distress

Soothe without Food

We saw earlier that one of the reasons we eat is because we need to soothe ourselves. How many times have you used caffeine and sodas to energize yourself during the day, hot soup and herbal teas to calm yourself down, or comfort foods to lift your mood? We all do these things from time to time and teach ourselves that eating is a way to soothe ourselves. To stop using food in unintended ways, we have to learn how to cope without using it.

In the chapter on stress, we discussed a few of those alternatives— slow breathing, deep muscle relaxation, closing your eyes and counting to ten, taking a time-out to refocus. Those same strategies work for emotional eating. When you feel anxious, take several deep breaths until you feel less tense. When you feel sad or lonely, take a hot bath, light candles, watch a funny movie, or read an inspirational book.

Think about what is comforting to you. Make a list of those comforting activities or things. Remember how I said music comforts me?

Not only do I like to listen to music, but playing the piano or flute brings me joy. When I need to relax, I play an instrument.

What are ways that you like to comfort yourself? Think of simple things that involve all the senses—lying down on a soft warm comforter, having a cup of tea, lighting candles that smell like fresh rain, dancing to your favorite music, watching a sunset, sitting out under the stars, rubbing lotion on your body, massaging your neck, or reading poetry, scriptures, or positive affirmations.

The goal is to soothe your soul without involving food. Once you practice comforting yourself without using food, you can practice tolerating discomfort. Food will no longer be needed to soothe you.

Think About the Pros and Cons

The Press Pause Principle is all about taking a moment to consider your options. If you are tempted to eat in response to emotions, you can run down a short pro-and-con checklist in your head or write it on a piece of paper. A list of pros and cons helps you stop and think before you act in ways you may regret later.

Ruby wants to eat because she is angry at her spouse. In the past, she ended an argument by going to the pantry and grabbing a bag of chips. This time, she decided to pause and write out a pro-and-con list. It looked like this:

PROS	CONS
If I eat, I will . . .	
Feel better immediately	The feeling is short lived, and I have the extra calories to deal with that will upset me later.
Distract myself with food	The distraction lasts only so long. The anger will return.
Feel momentary pleasure	I will also feel guilty because I wasn't hungry, add unnecessary calories, not solve the anger issue, and be upset with myself because this isn't helping me.

The cons win out when Ruby thinks through her decision to use food for emotional comfort. Her logical mind balances her emotions. Pressing *pause* gave her a chance to engage her logical mind in the middle of emotional distress and moderate it.

Improve the Moment

Being in the moment simply means we are aware of what is happening and attune to it before we respond. When we are *in* the moment instead of reacting *to* the moment, we can be intentional about our eating behavior.

Picture this scene. You are upset by a phone conversation you just had with your mother. You feel anxious and angry. You don't like this uneasiness but you cannot deal with it right now because you are at work and the phone call is over. There are doughnuts sitting by the coffeepot. Suddenly, you find yourself in front of the baker's dozen biting into a cream-filled confection.

Focus on the urge to eat. *Press pause* and take a deep breath. Focus your mind and tell yourself that this urge will pass if you wait it out. Push away negative thoughts about your mother because this is not something you can solve at this moment. Mentally, put a check mark on this conversation until you can deal with it later.

The mental check mark is important because you are not ignoring the fact that you are upset, but waiting for a better time to deal with the problem. You can't solve it immediately. Now, you have to wrap your brain around work and be present, feeling the upset and improving the moment.

Take another deep breath and encourage yourself to get back to work and deal with this later. Being upset is okay. But right now, you can't linger on that feeling. You know how to be assertive and will do so in a later conversation at home. You can resolve this issue with your mom. Right now, concentrate on what is before you—work.

Feel the upset, then mentally decide to handle it later and let it go for the time being.

Another way to improve the moment is to pray. Bill was anxious because he had to face his ex-wife at their daughter's vocal recital. When the two parents see each other, they usually argue.

As John's ex walked into the recital hall, he felt a sense of dread and mindlessly reached for the granola bar in his suit pocket. This time he decided to *press pause* and feel the dread. When he did, he released the tension in his jaw and face, took a deep breath, and prayed. *God, help me handle this as you would. Give me your peace. I am here for my daughter and want to enjoy it.*

When John shifted his attention to the moment and prayed for peace, he was able to let go of the dread and enjoy the recital. The music and his daughter were beautiful reminders of the good that came from his ex. For the moment, he sensed God's presence and his thoughts of the granola bar faded.

Tackle Your Emotions

Using emotional rescues to curb the urge to eat is a good strategy but ultimately we want to be able to manage our emotions directly. This usually requires facing emotions head-on and learning good interpersonal skills such as confrontation, assertiveness, and problem-solving.

So what happens when we allow ourselves to directly face uncomfortable emotions? Is it possible to feel the full intensity of any emotion, live through it, and come out fine in the end? Absolutely!

When an uncomfortable feeling hits, you may feel anxious and shaky and think, *I can't do this*, but you can. If you allow the feeling to unfold, you learn that you can get through it and survive your feelings without using food or distraction to ward them off. So let's talk about common feelings that we use food to medicate, and experiment with feeling them directly.

Dissipate Anxious Feelings

When we feel anxious, it affects us on all levels—physical, emotional, mental, behavioral, interpersonal, and spiritual. Because of this, we need ways to manage and eliminate anxiety to stay well.

We may think anxiety has no thought behind it. We just feel anxious and that feeling is overwhelming. But behind every anxious feeling is an anxious thought. Those anxious thoughts create and maintain anxious feelings—but only if we allow them to do so. The cure is to get at the anxious thought, situation, or issue that cues anxiety and then make changes.

The easiest way to eliminate anxiety is to eliminate the trigger. If anxiety is triggered by too much caffeine, cut back on caffeine. If the driver behind you makes you anxious, slow down and allow the person to pass. Stop smoking and your anxiety will lessen. Yes, you will still feel the effects of nicotine withdrawal, but don't confuse that with anxiety.

However, the reality is that you can't always eliminate the trigger. You may always have to deal with your unpleasant father-in-law. But you can learn how to release anxiety or not allow it to surface in the first place.

If your body is so tense you can't think, first relax your body using the breathing and muscle relaxation discussed on page 88. Then try to identify your thoughts. You will notice that they are usually negative, anticipating disaster or some negative outcome. You can change those thoughts to something encouraging and positive. For example, a typical anxious thought is, *What if . . .* You can change that to, *So what, I can handle this* or *I can get through this even though it won't feel good.*

In chapter 10, we talked about how changing the thought changes the feeling. Stop the anxious thought and replace it with encouragement and hope. In the case of the father-in-law, you stop the anxious thought by telling yourself, *I married his son, not him. This is how he is and I won't let it ruin my day.* Think of yourself like a life coach—someone who sees past the difficulty and focuses on the goal, which is to eliminate anxiety.

Another strategy is to embrace an anxious thought and stop fighting it. Let it come into your awareness, observe it, and let it go. You are not your thoughts. They come and go and are nothing more than experiences, as we learned in chapter 10. Review chapter 10 to work with anxious thoughts.

Release Your Sadness

One of the best ways to let go of sadness is to grieve. Years ago, when my brother was killed, I didn't grieve as much as I needed to right away. Instead of discharging the sadness through grief, I ate. When I was able to feel the loss deeply and release all the emotions associated with loss, I didn't need food to manage those feelings anymore.

The same was true when I experienced seven years of infertility. I had to grieve the possibility of never having children and trust that God knew what was best for me. Grieving releases the emotion of sadness. Trusting God turned the sadness into something tolerable. When I trust that God has not left me, forgotten about me, or stopped caring, I am confident that he will work on my behalf even when I see no evidence of this. This is what faith is—believing what we can't yet see.

Losses come in many forms, through death, divorce, illness, failed expectations, and lost dreams. Take the time to feel those losses. Cry, yell, scream out to God (he can handle it). Throw yourself on God's mercy and grace and allow him to take the loss and transform it for his glory.

Grieving a significant loss usually takes about two years. It is a process that can't be hurried or avoided without problems. During grief, you revisit different emotions multiple times. So anger may hit one day, sadness another. Allow yourself the opportunity to work through the emotions as they appear, and the urge to eat will lessen and eventually disappear.

Let Go of Anger

Anger is one of those emotions we need to learn to manage. People who say they don't get angry are in denial. Scripture speaks to the normalcy of getting angry when it tells us to be angry but not to sin. This means that anger is a natural part of our emotional makeup. However, the way we deal with anger is important. If we eat our way through it, we aren't coping in a good way.

And we need to understand that other people don't make us angry. We choose to be angry and we choose to sit on our anger or release it. So don't blame other people for anger issues. Focus instead on breaking the urge to eat in response to anger.

The first part to managing anger is to try to lower your physical and emotional arousal. You do this by employing relaxation exercises and taking charge of your thoughts. Getting enough sleep, exercising, eating well, and taking care of your body will also help you respond better to situations that make you angry.

The second part of anger management has to do with your thoughts. If you obsess about how unfair life is, refuse to acknowledge the fallibility of others, or hold unrealistic expectations of others or yourself, anger will be difficult to manage.

Life is unfair. We can't control how other people act. And people make mistakes. If you can accept these beliefs, you will be able to discharge anger more quickly than if you hold on to the illusion of controlling others or believe that life should always be fair. If your anger cannot be resolved, let it go anyway. Holding on to it will only lead to eating. Release anger so that it doesn't make you bitter or unforgiving. Both can be at the root of emotional eating.

Whenever you feel angry, pause, take several deep breaths, don't speak immediately, tell yourself to calm down and relax, count to ten if you need to, and then employ anger management strategies. They include learning to be assertive rather than aggressive (see chapter 14), calming down your body physically with a time-out or other relaxation exercise, talking out angry feelings with someone you can trust, and getting at the hurt behind anger and addressing that hurt or wounded area.

Avoid discharging your anger by hitting something, screaming, punching a bag or pillow, or throwing things. Researchers studying aggression at the University of Iowa[2] have discovered that ventilating anger in these ways only escalates it. On the other hand, you don't want to hold it in and suppress it because that can cause problems as well. Discharge anger with these guidelines found in Scripture:

- ▶ Stop and think.
- ▶ Get control over an angry thought and let it go.
- ▶ Be quick to listen, slow to speak.
- ▶ Don't give full vent to your anger.
- ▶ Don't get caught in name-calling.
- ▶ Don't take revenge.
- ▶ Forgive those who anger you.
- ▶ Get to the root of your anger.
- ▶ Don't stay angry.
- ▶ Give your anger over to God.
- ▶ Don't take offense.
- ▶ When possible, don't associate with angry people.

Fill the Loneliness or Boredom

The key to dealing with loneliness is to realize you are never really alone. God is always present. Even so, there are times when we crave the company of people. In those cases, we have to make the effort to get up and out.

Connecting with others takes effort and courage. It is not always easy to call someone or ask to do something with someone.

When I first moved to the Chicago area a few years ago, I missed my friends in Virginia. I really wanted to get to know the school moms in the new school my children attended. One day, I mustered up the courage to ask one of the moms to coffee. She said, "No offense, but my calendar is very full and I already have all the friends I need." Wow! That was a real eye-opener. But I chose not to take offense and to move on to someone I thought might be more receptive. I am really glad I didn't give up. Two women became my closest friends.

I had to make the effort to get out of my loneliness and have the courage to reach out. My first attempt wasn't exactly met with promise but I persevered, knowing the importance of having friends in my life. It may not always be easy, but don't give up. Eventually you will find people with whom you connect.

Beware of Excessive Fatigue

It has been a long day and you feel exhausted. You finally make it home and are greeted by two children who want to play, a dog wagging his tail, and a spouse looking for a few moments of kid relief. Everything in you wants to plop down on the couch and watch something mindless on TV. Since you can't do that, you reach for the leftover cake to give you energy. After all, you slept only five hours last night. You had to finish the board presentation that took you into the wee hours of the morning. Now you need a burst of energy to make it through the evening.

When we are tired, our defenses are down and we easily give in to urges to eat or cravings for particular foods. Running on empty is often a result of not getting enough sleep. Even though we need between seven and eight hours of sleep a night, few of us get those hours.

The best way to guard against tiredness is to set up good sleep habits and stick to them. Here are recommendations from the University of Maryland's Sleep Disorders Center.[3]

1. Try to stabilize your bedtime and time of awakening. The more scheduled both are, the better you do. Our bodies don't do well with different sleep and awakening times.

2. Try not to nap during the day. If you do, make it a short nap (thirty to forty-five minutes).

3. Don't have alcohol four to six hours before bedtime. It may seem like alcohol helps you sleep, but as the alcohol levels in your bloodstream fall, your body wakes up.

4. Don't have caffeine four to six hours before bedtime. Caffeine is a stimulant that keeps you awake and is found in coffee, sodas, chocolate, and other foods.

5. Avoid spicy, sugary foods.

6. Exercise, but do so at least two hours before bedtime.

7. Sleep on a comfortable bed.

8. Keep your bedroom at a comfortable temperature.

9. Keep the room dark and the noise to a minimum.

10. Make your bedroom an area for sleep and intimacy with your partner, not a place of other activity.

11. Light snacks such as a banana, warm milk, or herbal tea before bed may help you sleep.

12. Practice your relaxation exercises.

13. Try not to think about all the worries of the day. Get your mind on relaxing images.

14. Try a warm bath or engage in some other sleep ritual such as reading.

15. When you have trouble sleeping for more than half an hour, don't lie in bed and toss and turn. Get up and read until you are sleepy again.

The more you can prevent your body from getting tired, the easier it will be to pause and think before you eat. When you have the urge to eat in response to feeling tired, the solution is to take a brief nap or get to bed on time, not gobble chips and salsa!

Deal with Guilt and Shame

Guilt, if not handled properly, is one of those emotions that can trigger us to eat. Too many people can't get past the guilt once they confess their wrongdoing and ask for forgiveness. And some feel guilty for things they weren't even responsible for, such as being abused or having an unhappy mother.

So letting go of guilt requires two steps. First we have to determine if we did wrong. This means we must decide if we were responsible for a wrong act or if we are assuming responsibility that isn't ours. When we are guilty, confess the wrong, go to the one offended, and ask for forgiveness. Make sure you confess to God and not just people. It is God's forgiveness that releases us from the feeling of guilt.

The second part of releasing guilt requires us to let go of the confessed wrong. When we can't forgive ourselves, we are basically telling God that he is not big enough to take care of the issue. Thus, confession to God must include trusting him to forgive us and clear the slate. Sometimes it is easier to hang on to guilt because we can blame ourselves rather than deal with the uncertainty of relationships. Other times we might feel a need to punish ourselves.

If we cope with guilt by eating and then feel guilty when we eat, letting go of guilt requires self-forgiveness. Feeling guilty for eating only creates more guilt. Don't go there. Move on.

Guilt and shame are often linked together, but shame is very different from guilt. Guilt says, *I did something wrong*. Shame says, *I am bad*. Shame is personal and humiliating and serves no purpose but to leave you feeling worthless and wanting to eat.

Shari experienced feelings of shame that triggered her to eat. She put on pounds when she was a toddler and has been teased about her weight since then. With both of Shari's parents overweight, her family was known as "the fat people," and Shari felt shame from this most of her life.

Shari's childhood was unhappy because she was unable to do most of the activities in her physical education classes. At recess, she was called names or ignored. When Shari became a teenager, the teasing became unbearable. Shari retreated to the comfort of food and became depressed.

A dietitian began to work with Shari and show her how to eat in healthy ways. Shari wanted to lose weight but never was taught to eat healthfully. As Shari began to drop weight, her social life began to improve. However, the shame remained. Even though Shari eventually dropped more than a hundred pounds, she still saw herself as that pathetic fat kid whom everyone teased. Shari had changed her eating but needed to let go of the shame. Counseling helped Shari distinguish the shame she heaped upon herself from the shame others had bestowed on her. Once she recognized the difference, she was able to let go of both and view her body differently. Shari came to believe that her worth wasn't defined by how much she weighed.

Find a Substitute for Celebratory Eating

I mentioned at the beginning of this chapter that not all eating is in response to distress or uncomfortable feelings. Remember the survey indicating that 86 percent of people eat when happy?

Happy eaters eat when good things happen. They eat because they are influenced by family or friends or simply because they feel good and use food to celebrate happy feelings.

For them, overeating is all about food, love, family, community, and well-being. Happy eaters usually choose foods such as steaks and pizza over other comfort foods such as ice cream and chips.

You may be thinking, *I thought eating was supposed to be enjoyable.* It is, but there is a difference between enjoying what you eat and eating in response to an emotion. Food can bring happiness to a celebration. However, you don't want eating triggered every time you have a happy feeling. And sometimes we confuse feeling happy with being full.

So next time you feel happy because you found twenty dollars in your pocket, your son made the debate team, or your mother passed her real estate exam, celebrate in ways that don't involve food. Go to an event, buy a small gift, or take a break for a few hours. The goal is to find ways to celebrate your happiness that don't always involve food.

The bottom line is that we all eat in response to emotions from time to time. When we do, we need to lose the guilt and shame and simply acknowledge that we ate to pick up our mood or because we were happy. Our goal isn't to never eat in response to emotions. All-or-nothing thinking gets dieters in trouble.

What is important to remember is that emotional eating cannot become our main or only way to deal with feelings. We must learn other tools so that food doesn't become an emotional crutch.

Put together your list of emotional rescues to substitute for eating. Learn to soothe yourself with methods suggested, do a pro-and-con list, improve the moment, and tackle your emotions head on. All of these tools will expand your ability to cope with emotions and result in feeling more confident when it comes to mindful eating.

THE PRESS PAUSE PRINCIPLE

Plan to tolerate and manage emotions.

Attend to emotional triggers.

Understand ways to tolerate and manage your emotions that do not include eating.

Strategize ways to tolerate and manage emotions based on tools offered in this chapter.

Execute changes:
   ▷ Develop emotional rescues.
   ▷ Try soothing methods.
   ▷ Make a pro-and-con list.
   ▷ Improve the moment.
   ▷ Feel your emotions directly.

PAUSE FOR WISDOM
I count him brave who overcomes his desires
more than him who conquers his enemies,
for the hardest victory is the victory over self.
ARISTOTLE

13

RENEW YOUR MIND

I wish I could say that losing weight made all my food issues disappear. Somewhere in my imagination, I thought losing ten pounds would lead to contentment. It didn't. I still make poor choices with food. I fall off my eating plan and I return to my old habits of eating unconsciously. Changing this seems impossible. Yet somewhere inside me is this sense that I need more than my own efforts to shift my thinking. My own efforts seem to fail. As much and as hard as I try to think differently, I find myself stuck in old thoughts.

These reflections from a seasoned dieter bring to mind the issues we talked about in chapter 10: the power of the mind and how it influences eating. Our thoughts can help or hinder us when it comes to intentional eating. Yet making changes in how we think is difficult for many of us.

As we examine our thoughts, we notice the number and types of negative thoughts that invade our thinking. When it comes to food issues, typical negative thoughts involve failure to exercise self-control or giving in to mindless eating. This is not a happy way to live. Food thoughts should neither rule our day nor result in unnecessary guilt, shame, or even fear.

The question is how do we change our thoughts, especially if our experiences have been negative around food, dieting, and eating? How do we actually believe that eating can be a positive experience and stop struggling with food? How do we shift our negative thinking to positive?

The answers involve two strategies: refocus your view and renew your mind. Let's begin with refocusing. Refocusing involves changing your belief or view to allow for alternative ways to think. Too often our thinking gets stuck in a rut. We only view our problems or difficulties one way. Then, like the seasoned dieter, we feel trapped and unable to move forward.

Refocusing Your View

To better understand what refocusing means, think about taking photos. Let's say you are standing in front of a mountain landscape and decide to photograph it. When you look into the lens of the camera, your view of the landscape changes depending on the particular picture you take.

You can take a close-up photo of a bare section of the mountain. Based on that view, you might think the landscape is ugly. Or you could take a long shot and see the incredible colors and changes in terrain. A panoramic view would give even more depth and perspective to the scene. Or you could choose to focus on details in the foreground or background. Your specific focus determines the scene and creates different views depending on what you photographed. Basically, your focus determines your perception of that mountain.

Our minds involve focus and refocus. We can change our perception of food and eating by refocusing our view. Refocusing is simply taking a different picture from a different viewpoint of the same scene or situation. To refocus your thoughts means to think in a different way about an experience and place it in another frame. Can you interpret your experience from a different viewpoint?

Often you can't change a situation, but you can change how you think about it. And that is powerful. If you choose to think about food and eating from a positive view, it will change the way you feel and behave around food.

Food is a life-sustaining, nourishing substance available for our enjoyment. Embrace this positive view of food. Instead of thinking about food as the substance that makes us fat, refocus to think of food as the substance that sustains life. This refocus shifts your negative angle of thought to a positive one that provides a different view of food and eating. Our refocus is like taking a photo of the mountain from a specific perspective.

Here are more examples of refocusing food and eating thoughts:

ORIGINAL THOUGHT	REFOCUSED THOUGHT
I must deprive myself of foods I like.	I can eat foods I like but in moderation.
Eating is a struggle.	Eating is only a struggle if I make it one. It can be a delight.
I don't deserve to enjoy eating.	It is natural to enjoy food.
I am a bad person for eating candy.	Eating any food doesn't make me bad. My worth is not determined by food.
Losing weight will make me happy.	Happiness is about more than what I weigh.
I am weak willed when it comes to eating.	When I *press pause,* I can control what I eat.

When we refocus our eating thoughts from negative to positive, we are really just taking a new snapshot of an old scene and choosing to look at it differently. This fresh view has the power to move us forward, out of those stuck places of feeling failed and discouraged with our eating behavior. We can *press pause* and choose to think in a new way about our eating. We can look at any eating situation from a different angle with a positive focus. When we do this, positive feelings and behavior produce positive thoughts. Our minds calm down. Food is no longer the substance over which we struggle and eating becomes more pleasurable.

Courtney was obsessed with avoiding sugar. Whenever she "slipped" and ate something with sugar in it, she was convinced she would gain weight and she felt like a failure. Notice how Courtney's thought led to a negative feeling. But Courtney employed a refocus strategy to deal with her obsession. First she identified her negative thought. (*Eating sugar makes me fat and a failure*). Courtney's initial thought was not only negative but untrue. Eating sugar doesn't make someone automatically gain weight. What counts is how much sugar one eats in addition to other calories. Next she chose to refocus those thoughts to more positive and accurate thinking (*Sugar adds calories to what I eat but unless they add up to an extra 3,500 calories, I'm not going to gain even a pound, so I haven't failed*).

Ed also used refocus to change his eating habits. Ed's work requires him to travel. His thoughts about food and eating are reflected in this journal entry, which he willingly shares with us. His success had everything to do with refocus.

> *Whenever I get on a plane for a business trip, I begin the overeating process. I don't pay attention to my hunger because meals are a company expense. Something in me just kicks in and I feel almost obligated to eat everything that looks good. Usually this results in me feeling uncomfortably full and tired. Then I don't want to do any work, so mindless eating is fairly self-defeating.*
>
> *When I arrive at my location, I have to take clients out to dinner. Again, I splurge and overeat. In the past, that would have led to a pattern of overeating for the rest of my trip. Now, however, I realize that my overeating is prompted by my thinking. Because meals are free, I think I need to take advantage of the food. So you*

asked me to identify my negative food thought. This is it—if it's free, I need to eat it.

I grew up in a big family and money was always tight. I guess the fact that I can have whatever I want and not have to pay for it represents a type of freedom I've never had. But I'm excited to know that freedom also means I don't have to be a slave to the food. I've changed my thinking. I've refocused.

The food will always be there. I can access it anytime. More important is that I have learned to press pause and tune in to my body. I take a moment and ask, "Am I really hungry right now or am I eating because the food is free?" Instead of thinking I need to get all I can when I have the opportunity, I now think, I have the opportunity to eat what I want without worrying about the cost. I can be selective and dine according to my needs rather than my fears. This change in thinking has changed my eating habits. I no longer splurge and overeat. Now, I choose my food based on hunger and enjoy every bite, reminding myself how blessed I am to enjoy wonderful food and not have to pay for it.

When we examine our negative thoughts tied to food and eating, the challenge is to change our view to one that is more positive and more truthful. For years, I have worked with eating-disorder clients who will not believe the truth about their bodies and eating no matter how many times I have them repeat a different reality. This is especially true with body-image distortion. Telling an anorexic woman that she isn't fat doesn't change her reality. Her perception is that she is fat, despite her emaciated appearance.

One reason she hangs on to this distorted belief is because it is tied to deeper feelings about the self. Her body-image distortions won't change until she works through other negative and difficult areas of her life. In a strange way, the distortion feels protective. Even when she does work through life issues, she still must choose to change the way she sees her body by refocusing her thoughts. She has to be willing to embrace her body as part of her identity, but not the single defining source. She must practice self-care, believing in the importance of nourishing body, soul, and spirit in order to be whole. This action takes faith.

Having faith is usually the beginning of change—faith that her body and food can be her friend, faith that she can learn to face life struggles with help from others, and faith that she should become all she was intended to be.

However, there are times when lies and distortions in our thinking can be so implanted that refocusing isn't enough. Even when we force ourselves to think differently, we may not believe what we are thinking. When this is the case, we need a more comprehensive strategy. We need our minds renewed.

Renewing Your Mind

Mind renewing develops a positive relationship with food and eating. Why? Because without mind renewal, it is too easy to pair thoughts about food, weight, and eating with goodness or badness, and to listen to the distortions the culture presents us.

But what does it mean to renew our minds? Mind renewal is much more than reciting positive affirmations, although positive affirmations are involved. Positive affirmations are important but are usually our own attempts to fix our thinking, and the truth is that most of us need more than our own power or thinking to correct our thoughts when it comes to food and eating. We have too much history with the negative side of eating.

When positive affirmations include more than our own thoughts, they are much more powerful, and when they are drawn from what God has to say about us, they have the power to change and transform us if we choose to believe them. So, renewing the mind is a spiritual concept that involves exchanging our self-depreciating or negative thoughts for God's thoughts. It is how we silence the inner critic and learn to think about ourselves in a new way. It is not dependent on other people or past experiences. And it is not dependent on our own ability to manufacture positive thoughts.

Renewing the mind can become a daily activity that partners our natural mind with God's. The more we decide to line up our thoughts with God's way of thinking, the more hopeful, joyous, and peaceful we become. These outcomes require regular God encounters where we invite God to renovate our minds.

With the plethora of television shows on home renovation, it's not difficult for us to picture what a renovated mind might require—new construction, tearing down the old in favor of the new. A renewed mind is a changed mind.[1] In order to renovate my mind to God's, I must first have some understanding of how God thinks about me, food, and eating. This is so important because it is the counterbalance to how others think about me, how I may tend to think about myself, and the distortions I believe concerning food and eating that are embedded in the culture.

Let me explain. So often we develop a negative opinion of ourselves based on the hurtful and negative words of others. You may have been called a loser, lazy, weak willed, fat, unattractive, stubborn, or other insults. Those words penetrate the mind and often determine how we feel about ourselves, whether we realize it or not. The words of others, especially those with whom we are intimate, weigh much in determining our self-worth unless we have other words to counter those negative opinions. Add to this the cultural pressure to be thin and beautiful, and you have a recipe for negativity.

And even if we didn't have negative words spoken to us, we can manufacture negative thoughts about ourselves and eating in our own minds. Our minds are easily deceived and we are often blinded to the truth. It is easy to develop a negative picture of ourselves, others, and the culture if our minds are not constantly renewed with truth.

When we have strong desires to eat that have little to do with real hunger, our minds can become easily enticed by the emotion of the moment. We are tempted. Temptation tries to exploit our emotions, desires, and passions in a way that moves us away from the truth of our hunger and permits deception to rule. We tell ourselves we can't resist such deception. We allow the emotion of the moment to engage our thinking, which results in behavior we later regret.

Pressing *pause* allows us to stop and think about the moment. We can question our thought and decide if it is negative and if it is based on truth. This is the beauty of pausing. It gives us an opportunity to stop, think, and choose a new way to respond. In that short pause, we remind ourselves that negative thinking does not help us. Instead, we can replace our negative thought with a positive thought or affirmation. Here are a few suggestions for positive affirmations:

- *I am loved and worth loving.*
- *I determine what goes into my mouth.*
- *I am strong and can make good choices.*
- *Self-control is available to me from God.*
- *I can make good decisions.*

Take a few moments and come up with your own list based on your beliefs.

When God is with us, he helps us incline our emotions, desires, and passions to his will. We are confident that his power in us allows us to think clearly and make good decisions. But we have to be mindful of God's presence. The point is to stop looking at our circumstances and lives from our own limited perspective and to begin thinking about the strength we have through our relationship with God to overcome struggles and temptations. He is with us—a present help in times of trouble.

A Reason to Give Thanks

More than any other day of the year, Thanksgiving is a day devoted to eating. But one woman used this day of feasting to change her outlook toward food. She shares her journal entry:

It's Thanksgiving once again. In the past, I would have told you that my favorite thing about Thanksgiving was the food. All my life, this holiday has been all about the food. And I could always eat a large quantity of it in front of people and no one cared on this day! On Thanksgiving, everyone stuffs a turkey and themselves!

My entire focus on this holiday has always been about how well the food would turn out and what kinds of desserts would be served. I now understand that it wasn't bad to think about the festive foods. The problem was that it was my only focus for the holiday. I thought of nothing else. I spend this day with special people in my life but I never thought about them, the meaning of the holiday, only the food.

This year, things were different. My family got together and we enjoyed the meal. But for the first time, I also enjoyed playing games and being with friends. And for the first time, I focused on how blessed I am. I thanked God, my family, my friends for being in my life. Most of all, I was thankful for a renewed mind in which food thoughts didn't rule the holiday. What freedom that was! My eyes were opened to a new way to view Thanksgiving. Yes, the food was important and wonderful, but so were the people and the meaning of the holiday. I felt balance in my life for the first time. I am truly blessed.

The power of this journal entry is the shift in this woman's thinking. She is grateful for the holiday but has broadened her focus to include others. Freedom came when she dropped the negative thinking she used to pair with food and holidays. Now, she enjoys eating and being with her family. Positive affirmations help us be grateful for those things we may have taken for granted.

Turning Around Those Negative Thoughts

Whenever we encounter temptation or feel carried away by our emotions, it helps to *press pause* and remind ourselves of the times God has helped us in the past. Doing so builds our faith. When we feel defeated and overcome by food struggles, we can motivate ourselves by remembering the goodness in our lives.

We do have amazing strength to resist temptation, to think differently, and uncover lies. Near the end of the movie *The Matrix*, the character Neo realizes that he has control within the Matrix to stop bullets from enemy sources by simply saying *no*.

Like Neo, we have that same ability when it comes to negative thoughts. We say *no* to them and replace them with God's truth. This helps us live a life of self-control and abundance. So let's apply all of this to negative food thoughts. Identify negative thoughts and refuse to believe them. You have the power to change your beliefs and thoughts. Then apply the truth to thoughts of food: *Food is good for me; it sustains me; it is to be celebrated, enjoyed, and experienced as a delight.* Say *yes* to those thoughts. Let that truth sink deep into your spirit.

Then on a regular basis, review these positive thoughts in your head and choose to believe them. The more you believe a positive view of eating, the more you will lose automatic negative thoughts of food. Our beliefs inform our everyday thoughts.

Next, take any negative thoughts you have identified about food and eating and refocus them to a more positive view. Our confidence in being able to change our beliefs and thoughts can grow through believing in God and his promises. When we consistently encounter God in our lives, we affirm our beliefs. He tells us change is possible, that we can do all things through him.

Then take a few moments of your day to remember God's goodness to you. He is for you, not against you, and wants you to succeed at being more content with your life.

Finally, employ the strategy from chapter 10 regarding thoughts about eating certain foods: Instead of resisting food thoughts that come into our heads, allow them to come and go. Remember that research tells us that the more we resist thoughts of a specific food, the more we will eat it. Again, here is a chance to change your thinking. Remind yourself that they are only thoughts—not necessarily reality. Those thoughts that float through our brains about the hot fudge sundae tasting delicious or the french fries satisfying a craving are not a problem unless we begin to click on them. If we just let them be and don't struggle against them, eventually they will leave our minds. And while research can inform our beliefs, mind renewal transforms our thinking. A mind renewed by God's truth is a sound mind. The key is to take your negative thoughts, turn them over to God, and allow him to speak truth to your thoughts. Only God can transform our thinking.

There is great freedom in giving up negative thoughts about food and eating. Approaching each day with a sense of thankfulness for the food you have and the choices before you will lift your spirits and bring a new appreciation for life. A renewed mind takes the struggle out of eating.

THE PRESS PAUSE PRINCIPLE

Plan to develop positive beliefs about food and eating.

Attend to your negative thoughts and self-efforts.

Understand that when influenced by others, our own thoughts, and our culture, thinking can easily become negative. We are susceptible to lies and distortions in our food thoughts and need to replace them with more positive, truthful thoughts.

Strategize ways to change your thinking and actually have it transformed.

Execute changes:
  ▷ Refocus your view and renew your mind.
  ▷ Exchange your negative thoughts for God's truth.

PAUSE FOR WISDOM

Eating is not merely a material pleasure. Eating well gives a spectacular joy to life and contributes immensely to goodwill and happy companionship. It is of great importance to the morale.

ELSA SCHIAPARELLI

14

EATING WITH PEOPLE, NOT BECAUSE OF THEM

The better and more confident you are at handling yourself around others, the less likely you will be to eat in response to relationship issues. Too often, we eat our way through frustration with a mother-in-law, disappointment with a boss, or rejection from a friend.

As we learned in a previous chapter, our emotions can prompt unintentional eating. And one main source of emotions is our intimate and interpersonal relationships. So we need to develop effective ways to handle them. When we address relationship issues in healthy ways, our relationships can improve and we no longer need to eat in an attempt to take away bad feelings.

So think about your relationships and the triggers that lead you to eat. When the trigger occurs, respond with a new action instead of eating. Repeat that new action until it feels familiar and comfortable. Over time, you will break the connection between the trigger and eating. And you will learn how to be more effective with the people you encounter.

One of your triggers might be eating after an argument with your spouse. Before the next argument occurs, decide what you could do instead of going to the pantry and eating due to frustration. Perhaps you could take a brief time-out and calm down, using the deep breathing exercises on page 88. Then, when you are calmer, employ conflict-resolution skills to the argument. Refuse to go to the refrigerator and eat.

I would suggest beginning with one relationship trigger at a time. Sometimes it helps to face the worse problem first, or work on a trigger that is a high priority or will have the biggest impact. When choosing a trigger, try to focus more on the facts of the moment than on fault finding, blaming, feeling guilt, shame, or some other negative thought or emotion. Observe the thought or feeling associated with a trigger and then behave in a new way.

When you argue with your spouse, you may feel upset. That's okay. Allow yourself to feel upset. Tell yourself that this is only an argument and that you need to calm down. Practice relaxation. Apologize to your spouse for approaching the problem in an angry manner and ask if the two of you can discuss the problem without getting into a fight. Then confront the problem with the new set of skills you'll learn in this chapter.

The more you practice a new pattern of behavior, the more confident you will feel in terms of resolving issues. Then you won't need to turn to food out of frustration.

Keep in mind that any time we change an old pattern of behavior, we usually feel tense and unsure of ourselves. Change means letting go of the familiar and doing something unfamiliar. Whenever we do something unfamiliar, it feels uncomfortable at first. Eventually we get better at this new behavior and it becomes habit.

Change What You're Saying to Yourself

Angela's boss bothers her. He rarely has good things to say and loves to dish out criticism. One afternoon when he stopped at Angela's cubicle and made negative comments about her work, just the sight of him made her cringe; she calmed herself down with the chocolate stashed in her top desk drawer. After months of complaining about how angry her boss made her feel, Angela decided to change her reaction to him.

Angela felt harassed by her boss because his criticism was undeserved. She considered confronting him but had witnessed several of her colleagues try this tactic, with bad outcomes. Angela's boss was not open to feedback and punished people who confronted him. Thus Angela felt stuck and couldn't figure out any way to calm down other than eating, although she knew that eating wasn't helping matters in the long run. Then she realized she could change how she felt about her boss's criticism. Instead of becoming livid at his insensitivity and unkind remarks every day, Angela accepted the fact that she couldn't change her boss. He seemed to enjoy putting down others and showed no evidence of changing. She could change jobs, which she didn't want to do, or accept the situation. She chose the latter and decided to change how she felt about her boss's behavior. Here's what she did.

The next time the boss approached her cubicle and belittled her work, Angela paused and used self-talk—the internal dialogue we have with ourselves. Since Angela didn't believe her boss's comments were fair, she refused to take him seriously, knowing he had no credibility. Her self-talk went like this: *My boss is negative. His comments are not based on any real evaluation. I know I did a great job on this assignment and I refuse to allow his comment to ruin my day. I'll just pat myself on the back and move on.* When she changed her self-talk, her feelings changed. She was no longer so angry and the urge to eat subsided.

Angela employed a useful strategy in life: Change what you can and accept what you cannot change. In this case, she could change the way she felt about her boss by thinking differently about him. Her self-talk changed from how much she disliked him to how little credibility he really had. She learned to ignore his undeserved criticism and refused to allow him to ruin her day.

Changing how you feel typically changes how you behave. In Angela's case, she stopped her mindless eating. Changing her self-talk was not as easy as eating her anger away, but it was much more productive in the long run. It gave Angela the power to control her emotions and thoughts and didn't allow someone else to determine her mood. And her self-talk was the key to breaking the habit of unintentional eating.

Confront the Problem Head-On

If you are thinking, *I'm not very good at confrontation and the idea of confronting people instead of eating is a bit daunting to me,* you are in good company. Most of us have problems confronting anyone, or else do it in a too-aggressive manner.

For many of us, fear keeps us from healthy confrontation. Based on our childhood learning, our life experiences, and the potential to create more conflict, we often avoid conflict because we don't believe the outcome will be good.

Our tendency is to blame others or make excuses for our behavior when confrontation occurs. However, blame doesn't resolve anything and triggers us to eat.

Furthermore, when we do muster up the courage to confront someone, we don't typically receive a thank-you or grateful response. Nevertheless, it is the heart of God that we learn to confront each other in love. Scripture provides guidance in this area. The Apostle Paul talks about discord and encourages conflict resolution by telling the church in Corinth, "God has called us to peace" (1 Corinthians

7:15 NASB). This is also true for today. But to live in peace often means we must engage in healthy confrontation.

Healthy confrontation is done in love. It is characterized by mercy and forgiveness. The more you can approach someone with love and be ready to forgive with mercy, the better your chances of lowering the person's defenses and resolving the issue.

Once you have the right spirit behind confrontation, you can practice the skill. When you decide to confront someone, know the facts and do not respond only to emotions. Then focus the confrontation on one point, not a host of grievances. Avoid judging or accusing the person. Listen to what they say and paraphrase it out loud to check your understanding. Finally see if a positive action is possible. Try to resolve the issue and move on.

If you think you need to confront someone, ask yourself this question first: *Is this a battle I need to fight?* Sometimes we can choose to let go of an issue and move on without it bothering us. We don't need to confront every issue that creates potential conflict. Confront those specific issues that trigger overeating or unintentional eating.

The more you practice healthy confrontation, driven by the right motives, the urge to eat will diminish over time. And the more you practice, the easier it will be to address issues directly and resolve them.

Verbalize Your Worries

I can't tell you how many people I have treated who eat because they haven't learned to use their voices and speak up. They muffle their thoughts and feelings by eating instead of talking.

Some people take on too much and don't learn to say no to requests. Then they are secretly angry and feel stressed, which results in eating. What can you do? Don't agree to one more school-mom activity that puts you over the edge! Don't volunteer in church because no one else agrees to take on another responsibility! Learn to say no and not feel guilty. You *have* to set boundaries or you will eat out of frustration and irritation.

Others are afraid to speak up because they have not been encouraged to do so in the past or were punished for being assertive. This usually leads to keeping your mouth shut when it comes to speaking up but opening it for food!

Still others feel they must please people, so they don't speak up, and eat instead. Once you understand the connection between non-assertive behavior and eating, asserting yourself is a way to break the behavior. Developing assertiveness skills keeps you from giving in to things you really don't want to do. It also prevents anger buildup and aggression. It is a practiced skill that helps you manage your relationships.

The first step to being assertive is to know what it is that you want. Usually we know what doesn't feel good or what we don't like, but we don't always know what we want. It takes some thought to figure out what it is you need and to verbalize it. You may fear that other people may not agree to meet your need. But don't let that stop you from asserting your needs.

The second step to assertiveness is to open your mouth and speak. If you don't speak up, you may never get your needs met. Don't expect other people, especially spouses, to read minds. To give them a chance to respond, you have to tell others what you need or want or what you are unhappy about.

Becoming more assertive is not difficult once you believe it will be helpful in your relationships. If you are calm and practice, you'll become more comfortable. When you address problems as they occur, you won't build up anger and hold on to things that can grow into resentment. A lack of assertiveness can be a root of depression, anxiety, and eating disorders.

Assertiveness Can Change Your Life

When you practice being assertive, you not only improve your physical and psychological health but also gain respect. People may not like what you have to say all the time, but most will respect you for speaking your mind.

Erin used assertiveness to help her troubled marriage. She was lonely in her marriage but decided to focus on her behavior rather than her feelings. When she did, her feelings for her husband changed. Here is what she did.

Erin and her husband rarely did anything together and her husband said very little at home. Instead, he busied himself with television, video games, or home projects. Erin tried to make conversation, but he avoided her as much as possible.

The loneliness drove Erin to eat. She realized something had to change because she was gaining weight and felt lonely. Erin decided to speak up, but in a way that was different from the past. In the past, her attempts to be assertive were all about criticizing her husband and pointing out his flaws. When she did these things, her husband became defensive and became even quieter.

So Erin changed her tactics. Instead of criticizing her husband's lack of interaction or talking, she refocused her conversation. She talked about how lonely and empty she felt. As she focused more on her feelings, her husband began to listen. Erin was not criticizing him but simply reflecting her wish to have more time to do things together. This got her husband's attention.

Erin told her husband that she was eating so much because she felt empty and was desperate for a friend. To her surprise, her husband felt the same. He used media to escape his loneliness. The two agreed to go to marriage counseling because neither was getting their friendship needs met in the marriage. The hope was that they could restore what they somehow had lost over the years. They used to have fun together and share their dreams.

Erin's decision to be assertive about her *own* feelings rather than criticize her husband helped move things in the right direction. And her urge to eat diminished because she was addressing a problem she had numbed with food.

To move the relationship in a more positive direction, Erin had to stop using food as a way to cope with interpersonal distress and try something new. Becoming assertive didn't cause defensiveness. It opened the door for better communication.

But realize that when you stop using food to distract, soothe, or numb yourself, you have to replace the food with something else. In too many instances, people give up food but try alcohol, drugs, shopping, or some other addictive and damaging behavior. Plan ahead and develop a list of activities or actions you will turn to instead of eating.

Solve Issues, Don't Eat Over Them

Once you commit to the idea of confronting interpersonal issues and learn to be more assertive, you can use the conflict management skills discussed later in this chapter to help you solve relationship problems. Then you can turn conflict into opportunities to increase your intimacy with people you care about.

Conflict is a normal part of life. People don't always agree with our needs or goals. They think differently than we do and have different values. When people clash with our point of view, it results in conflict. For instance, your boss may not see the futility of giving you a task that you feel is a colossal waste of time. The teacher may disagree with how you did your assignment. Your spouse may disagree with you on a parenting issue.

Furthermore, people do not always do what they say they will do or do it to our satisfaction. And there are times where we don't agree with the way people behave or think. In an ideal world, people would always behave politely, show concern for others, be true to their word, and follow through with what they say they will do. Unfortunately, we don't live in that world.

During any given day, multiple opportunities occur to engage in conflict with people. How we deal with conflict is what matters. When conflict creates a source of stress, we have to be careful not to use food to calm us down. Remember two important approaches to reduce stress:

- ▸ Deal with conflict and try to resolve it.
- ▸ Make your expectations realistic.

Alter your expectations. Sam had a boss who constantly challenged his decisions. Sam was not very assertive and felt anxious every time this happened, and reached for the candy stored in his desk. Sam needed to work on his assertiveness skills but realized that his boss made final decisions. Here's how Sam changed his expectations: *It's annoying and frustrating when my boss challenges every decision I make, but it's part of my job. I either accept it, asserting myself where I can, or look for a new job.* Sam stopped eating his stashed candy once he altered his expectations.

Find a realistic solution. Louise was stressed by her husband's poor financial planning. Based on her childhood experience, she expected her husband to be in charge of finances. That's what her father had done and he was good at it. Louise's husband was not. Holding on to unrealistic expectations left Louise irritated and stressed. She mindlessly ate until she realized the source of her stress: her husband didn't meet her expectations.

Louise couldn't change her husband, but she could change her expectations and make them more realistic. After years of nagging her husband to do better, Louise finally decided financial planning was not his gift and that she needed to be more involved. Fortunately, her dad had taught her much about balancing accounts and running a household. Louise took over the finances and let go of her unrealistic hope that her husband would eventually blossom into a financial planner. Once Louise adjusted her expectations, she stopped stress-eating.

Change behavior that results in eating. As a young adult, Rebecca wanted to be independent but had trouble separating herself from Mom. She checked every decision with her mother. For example, Rebecca knows how to pay her bills but checked with her mother whenever she wrote a check—and after the conversation, she found herself eating cookies from her pantry.

Rebecca began to examine the relationship with her mother as a possible trigger for unintentional eating. Rebecca knew that she was too dependent on her mom. She figured out that her unintentional eating was related to her inability to break this dependence and function more autonomously.

Once Rebecca decided to make decisions on her own, her unintentional eating stopped. Making independent decisions brought a certain level of anxiety, but she felt more confident and in charge of her life. That newfound confidence was enough to stop her anxious eating.

At times, we need to evaluate our expectations, perhaps readjust them, or simply let them go. *Press pause*, take a deep breath, and ask, *Is this an expectation that is realistic or even worth stressing out over?* If not, let it go and adjust your thinking. The more accepting and forgiving we are of other people's shortcomings, the better we handle life. The more realistic our expectations are, the less stress we bring upon ourselves.

Dealing with Conflict in Marriage

Marriage can be a major source of conflict. From studies on marital conflict cited in *The Family Therapy Networker*,[1] we know that men become more physiologically aroused during fights than women, with higher blood pressure and heart rate. And they stay upset longer than women after a fight is over.

This means that both men and women need to know how to effectively deal with conflict in marital situations. Men need to pace themselves and be aware of their physical reactions. They need to slow down the overwhelming physical responses by calming themselves. Women need to be aware of the physical responses men are experiencing, and understand why it might take men longer to calm down.

Instead of using food to de-stress after an argument, couples can take a brief time-out (twenty-five to thirty minutes) when conflict begins to heat up. During the time-out, relax the body by taking deep breaths while stopping negative thoughts about the other person. This is very important when a fight occurs.

If you pause but continue to think negative thoughts about your partner, you will remain tense. Instead, refocus your thoughts on something positive about your spouse like, *This is the woman I married who loves me. We can work this out.* Or, *I know we are both upset right now but this conflict can be resolved. Calm down. We can do this.* Once calm, go back to your spouse and use conflict-resolution skills to resolve the issue. The point is to monitor your stress during the conflict and do what you can to reduce that stress in order to prevent a food run after a fight.

Remember, conflict-resolution skills include calming yourself down using techniques such as taking a brief time-out, deep breathing, or counting to ten before tackling the issue. We listen better when we aren't angry or defensive. Try to understand what the other person is saying or needs. If you can get at the real need behind a conflict, you will go further in resolving it than if you are looking to be right or to win.

To resolve a conflict, choose a time when neither of you are angry or argumentative. Be respectful when discussing your point of view. Be clear about the problem. Use "I" statements rather than accusatory sentences. "I" statements verbalize how you feel and focus on the behavior at hand rather than the person. Listen to what the person has to say without interrupting him or her. Try to put yourself in his or her position and see the issue from his or her point of view. Give ideas on how to solve the problem and talk through the consequences of each alternative. Agree on a solution you can both live with and one that works. Check on the solution after you've implemented it to see if it is working.

In dealing with relationship conflict, remind yourself that the other person probably has a different view of the problem. This isn't a bad thing. It just means that your first step is to try and understand where that person is coming from—what is his or her perspective? To gain perspective, try to listen carefully. Don't interrupt. The goal is to understand the other person, not get your point across. You will eventually get your turn to be understood.

When you tackle a conflict, it also helps to have ground rules. These include:

▶ No name-calling
▶ No hurtful comments
▶ No cynical remarks
▶ No threats
▶ No vague statements
▶ Respectful communication
▶ Focusing on one issue at a time

▶ Using "I" statements instead of blame
▶ Not making assumptions

Now you may be thinking that this sounds like a lot of work. Eating is much easier than going through all those steps! True, but eating doesn't solve your problems. It only compounds them.

Our reluctance to deal with conflict is often based in fear of rejection. No one likes to be rejected, and because so many people have poor conflict-resolution skills, rejection is a possible outcome. Even so, your relationships will not grow closer with conflict avoidance.

The other hesitancy that comes with addressing conflict is that we may have to take responsibility for change. After all, if you bring up an issue, it may require you to do something different in order to solve it. This means *you* might have to change. But again, the outcome is worth it. Taking responsibility for change usually means your relationship will grow stronger.

Resolving conflicts requires you to use problem-solving skills. In problem-solving you state the problem, look for areas of agreement, explore new ideas, try a solution, and evaluate the chosen solution.

All healthy relationships need this kind of cooperation and compromise in order to increase intimacy and keep relationships strong. And if we want to be effective in our relationships and not use food to cope with conflicts, these are important skills to practice.

THE PRESS PAUSE PRINCIPLE

Purpose to resolve relationship issues and not eat because of them.

Attend to those relationship conflicts that cue mindless eating.

Understand the importance of developing effective ways to address relationship conflicts and frustrations.

Strategize ways to be more effective in resolving conflict.

Execute changes:
> ▷ Accept what you can't change and change what you can.
> ▷ Change your self-talk.
> ▷ Change your reaction.
> ▷ Confront problems.
> ▷ Assert yourself in your intimate relationships.
> ▷ Use conflict-resolution skills and problem-solving.

PAUSE FOR WISDOM
We should look for someone to eat and drink with before looking for something to eat and drink.
EPICURUS

PART FIVE

EXECUTE

To execute means to completely put into effect a plan. The key to executing and sustaining change involves taking action—purpose to pause, attend to the moment, understand why you do what you do, strategize change, and then implement what is required to become an intentional eater.

Now that you fully understand the Press Pause Principle, it is time to take action.

Execution of a plan is usually where people fall short. They plan, pay attention, understand, and even develop strategies, but then fail to do what they set out to do. And execution is what counts. No one wants to become one of those well-intentioned people who knows what works but just doesn't do it.

This last section provides ten guidelines that will help you execute change. Can we move forward and use what we know to become an intentional eater? We have the cure, but will we take advantage of it? Execution is about doing!

15

PRESS PAUSE
AS A LIFETIME PRACTICE

You are armed with what you need to become an intentional eater. You have the awareness you need when it comes to food and eating. Now it is up to you to put it all into practice, a moment at a time.

These ten guidelines will help you execute the *pause*. You can reach the goal of saying good-bye to mindless eating and hello to joyful eating. You now know the secret to having a positive relationship with food.

1. Stay Honest

When it comes to pausing and examining how you think and feel, stay honest. Honesty will keep you from fooling yourself and living in denial. Lose whatever pity or blame you might be tempted to engage in and be authentic. The more you learn about your eating habits, the easier it will be to make those strategic changes listed at the end of each chapter. But you have to be honest about your shortcomings and areas that need change.

2. Stay in Relationships

Even though *press pause* is about stopping, quieting your mind, and observing your thoughts and actions, it is dangerous to isolate yourself from others. While silence is highly valued and needed in our crazy busy lives, it is in the context of relationships that we grow and sharpen one another. We need one another to live intentional lives. Other people provide us with a much-needed perspective on our behavior. And the support we receive from others is often the motivation we need to keep moving forward. Value your relationships and work at them.

3. Stay Energized

It is easy to give up and give in. Change is tiring and takes work. This is why people hang on to old patterns of behavior even when they don't work. It is easy to become complacent. Keep up your energy level by renewing your mind daily and not giving in to complacency.

4. Stay Focused

To not lose sight of the goal, we must keep our focus. Throughout this book, I have reminded you of the goal: to become an intentional eater and enjoy eating. Stay focused and you will reach this goal.

5. Stay Strong and Uncompromised

Intentional eaters don't compromise what they know works. It may be easier to live mindlessly, but in the long run, it won't satisfy or bring lasting peace. We *press pause* and consider why we are eating although it would be easier to rush through a meal and not think about it. Eating thoughtlessly once in a while is normal, but when mindlessness becomes a pattern, you are compromising the *pause*. Stay strong in your resolve to do what you know works.

6. Stay Sane

Don't allow the crazy and defeating thoughts of our culture to rule your mind. There is so much talk of dieting and fad eating that we can find ourselves thinking crazy thoughts about food and our bodies. Stay sane by renewing your mind and refocusing on what you know to be true.

7. Stay Present

Living with past failures and wondering if you can be effective in the future takes you nowhere. Stay in the present and focus on the moment. Every moment is a new opportunity for success.

8. Stay Forgiving

We all make mistakes. There will be days in which we hurry and eat unintentionally. If you can forgive and exercise grace, you can begin each moment anew.

9. Stay Centered

Your spiritual life is what keeps you centered. Practice spiritual disciplines and meditate on God and his word. This is what gives you the power to do what you need to do.

10. Stay Positive

You can do this. You can *press pause* before you eat and become an intentional eater. None of this is too difficult to apply if you are willing to take a few moments to change.

PAUSE FOR WISDOM
Nobody can go back and start a new beginning, but anyone can start today and make a new ending.
MARIA ROBINSON

ACKNOWLEDGMENTS

Writing a book is a time-consuming process made possible only by my supportive family. Many thanks go to the other Dr. Mintle, Norm: you provided loving care and picked up the slack when I locked myself away to write in the home office for hours on end. Thanks also to my teens, Matt and Katie: once again, you both understood the commitment of time I needed and evidenced sensitive hearts and sweet spirits. And to my puppy, Zoe: thank goodness you required me to get off the computer and take you for daily walks. I don't know what shape my back would be in without your cute little face urging me to the marsh.

I thank my new family at Howard Books for picking up the vision and making this book a reality. Cindy Lambert for not giving up, pursuing me with such grace and providing thoughtful editing; Susan Wilson for her vigilance with details; and Greg Petree, Melissa Teutsch, and Kristy Myers for their vibrancy and vision in marketing and publicity. Thanks also to Sara Henry and Jennifer Greenstein for their insight and feedback during the early stages of my manuscript.

Finally, I thank my extended family, who taught me the joy of eating and shared their love of home-cooked meals and huge family gatherings. These are memories I will always cherish.

NOTES

1: Press Pause: It Takes Only a Moment

1. William Ira Bennett, "Beyond Overeating," *The New England Journal of Medicine* 332, no. 10 (1995): 673–74; R. L. Weinsier et al., "Do Adaptive Changes in Metabolic Rate Favour Weight Gain in Weight-Reduced Individuals? An Examination of the Set-Point Theory," *The American Journal of Clinical Nutrition* 72 (2000): 1088–94.
2. F. Grodstein, R. Levine, L. Troy, T. Spencer, G. A. Colditz, and M. J. Stampfer, "Three-Year Follow-up of Participants in a Commercial Weight-Loss Program. Can You Keep It Off?" *Archives of Internal Medicine* 156 (1996): 1302–06.

2: Hurry Up to Slow Down

1. Food Navigator, " 'Flexi-eating'—the Future for Food Consumption?" (May 23, 2002). Retrieved from http://www.foodnavigator.com/Science-Nutrition/Flexi-eating-the-future-for-food-consumption.
2. Ibid.

3. Health 24, "Breakfast—the Most Frequently Missed Meal." Retrieved online October 21, 2007, from http://www.health24.com/dietnfood/General/15-742-775, 18362.asp.

4. Pew Research Center, "Who's Feeling Rushed." Retrieved online from http://pewresearch.org/social/pack.php?PackID=2.

5. *The KJV New Testament Greek Lexicon.* Retrieved online October 9, 2006, from http://bible.crosswalk.com/Lexicons/Greek/grk .cgi?number=3115&version=kjv.

6. CASA 2000 Teen Survey, "Teens with 'Hands-Off' Parents at Four Times Greater Risk of Smoking, Drinking, and Using Illegal Drugs as Teens with 'Hands-On' Parents," *Columbia News* (October 1, 2002).

7. CASA, "Why Family Day?" *Columbia News* (September 1, 2002).

8. M. W. Gillman, S. L. Rifas-Shiman, A. L. Frazier, H. R. H. Rockette, C. A. Camargo, A. E. Field, C. S. Berkey, and G. A. Colditz, "Family Dinners and Diet Quality among Older Children and Adolescents," *Archives of Family Medicine* (2000): 9235–240. A questionnaire using 24-hour recall that was mailed to children of participants in the ongoing Nurses' Health Study II. Retrieved online October 6, 2004, from http://216.239.41.104/search?q=cache:H5jg_Q0v74J:edprojects.che.umn.edu/take back/downloads/research.pdf+overscheduled+kids+and+under connected+families&hl=en.

9. Sandra L. Hofferth, "Changes in American Children's Time, 1981–1997," University of Michigan's Institute for Social Research, center survey (January 1999). National probability samples of American families with children ages 3–12, using time diary data from 1981 and 1997. Findings on how time use is associated with children's well-being are reported in S. L. Hofferth, "How American Children Spend Their Time," *Journal of Marriage and the Family* 63 (2001): 295–308. Retrieved online October 4, 2004, from http://216.239.41.104/search?q=cache:H5jg _Q0-v74J:edprojects.che.umn.edu/takeback/downloads/research

.pdf+overscheduled+kids+and+underconnected+families&
hl=en.

10. D. DeNoon, "Future-Is-Now Attitude Blamed for Obesity,"
WebMD Medical News (March 17, 2004). Retrieved online August 21, 2006, from http://www.webmd.com/content/article/84/97989.htm.

3: Listen to Your Body Talk

1. Sharron Dalton, *Our Overweight Children: What Parents, Schools and Communities Can Do to Control the Fatness Epidemic* (Berkeley, CA: University of California Press, 2005), 49.

2. J. Kluger, "The Science of Appetite," *Time* (June 11, 2007): 49–62.

3. "Does Ice Water Burn More Calories? How Stuff Works." Retrieved online July 23, 2007, from http://health.howstuffworks.com/question447.htm.

4. Kluger, "The Science of Appetite."

5. J. E. Blundell, S. Goodson, and J. C. G. Halford, "Regulation of Appetite: Role of Leptin in Signaling Systems for Drive and Satiety," *International Journal of Obesity* 1, suppl. 1: S29–S34.

6. Elaine Magee, "How to Stop Overeating." Retrieved online August 20, 2007, from http://men.webmd.com/guide/overcoming-overeating.

7. Science Daily, "Bottoms Up: Purdue Study Links Beverages to Weight Gain," Purdue University (November 23, 1998). Retrieved online July 22, 2007, from http://www.sciencedaily.com/releases/1998/11/981123080917.htm.

8. Magee, "How to Stop Overeating."

9. Kluger, "The Science of Appetite."

10. Rachael Heller and Richard Heller, *The Carbohydrate Addict's Diet: The Lifelong Solution to Yo-Yo Dieting* (New York: Signet Books, 1993).

4: From Impulsive to Thoughtful

1. Lisa Mancino and Jean Kinsey, "Diet Quality and Calories Consumed: The Impact of Being Hungrier, Busier, and Eating Out," working paper 04-02, The Food Industry Center, University of Minnesota (March 2004), *Choices* (Fall 2002). Retrieved online October 1, 2007, from http://agecon.lib.umn.edu/cgi-bin/pdf_view.pl?paperid=13657&ftype=.pdf.

2. Brian Wansink, *Mindless Eating* (New York: Bantam, 2007), 79–80.

3. Steve Bradt, "Brain Takes Itself On over Immediate vs. Delayed Gratification," *Harvard Gazette* (October 21, 2004). Retrieved online September 25, 2007, from http://www.hno.harvard.edu/gazette/2004/10.21/07-brainbattle.html.

4. Y. Shoda, W. Mischel, and P. K. Peake, "Predicting Adolescent Cognitive and Social Competence from Preschool Delay of Gratification: Identifying Diagnostic Conditions," *Developmental Psychology* 26 (1990): 978–86.

5. R. Baumeister, T. Heatherton, and D. Tice, *Losing Control: How and Why People Fail at Self-Regulation* (San Diego, CA: Academic Press, 1994).

6. Lisa Mancino and Jean Kinsey, "The Road to Not-So-Wellville: Paved with Good Intentions and Misperceptions—Diet Choices," *Choices* (Fall 2002). Retrieved online October 1, 2007, from http://findarticles.com/p/articles/mi_m0HIC/is_4_17/ai_100755074/pg_3.

7. As quoted in *Perilous Pursuits*, Joseph M. Stowell (Chicago: Moody Press, 1994), 47.

5: The Many Meanings of Food

1. CNN Interactive, "The Food of Kwanzaa" (1996). Retrieved online April 14, 2007, from http://www.cnn.com/EVENTS/1996/kwanzaa/food.html.

2. "Hispanic-American Influence on the US Food Industry," selected references prepared in commemoration of the USDA Hispanic Heritage Month Celebration (September 15–October 15, 2002). Retrieved online April 14, 2007, from http://www.nal.usda.gov/outreach/HFood.html.

3. "Cultural Diversity: Eating in America—Asian," Ohio State University Extension Fact Sheet. Retrieved online April 16, 2007, from http://ohioline.osu.edu/hyg-fact/5000/5253.html.

4. Better Health Channel, "Food and Celebrations," RMIT University Department of Food Science. Retrieved online February 28, 2007, from http://www.betterhealth.vic.gov.au/bhcv2/bhcarticles.nsf/pages/Food_and_celebrations?OpenDocument.

6: Relax and Put Down the Fork

1. Rodrique Ngowi, "Holiday Stress Pushing More Women to Comfort Eat, Study Shows," Associated Press (December 17, 2006). Retrieved online May 15, 2007, from http://www.boston.com/news/local/rhode_island/articles/2006/12/17/holiday_stress_pushing_more_women_to_comfort_eating_study_shows/.

2. B. Wansink, M. Cheney, and N. Chan, "Exploring Comfort Food Preferences across Gender and Age," *Physiology and Behavior* 79, nos. 4–5 (September 2003): 739–47.

3. Kirsten Galisson, "Food for Comfort," *Psychology Today* (January/February 2001). Retrieved online March 5, 2007, from http://www.psychologytoday.com/articles/pto-20010101-000021.html.

4. Science Daily, "Comfort-Food Cravings May Be Body's Attempt to Put Brake on Chronic Stress," University of California–San Francisco (September 11, 2003). Retrieved online March 5, 2007, from http://www.sciencedaily.com/releases/2003/09/030911072109.htm.

5. "Gender Preferences in 'Comfort' Foods Stem from Childhood," University of Illinois at Urbana–Champaign (July 2, 2003). Re-

trieved online May 15, 2007, from http://www.eurekalert.org/pub
_releases/2003-07/uoia-gpi070203.php.

6. Linda Myers, "Comfort Foods Help Women When They're Blue,
but Increase Male Highs, Study Finds," *Chronicle Online*, Cornell
University (November 15, 2005). Retrieved online May 15, 2007,
from http://www.news.cornell.edu/stories/Nov05/LeBel.comfort
.food.lm.html.

7. T. Koepke, "Caffeine's Effects Are Long-Lasting and Compound
Stress," DukeHealth.org (2002). Retrieved online August 6, 2007,
from http://www.dukemednews.org/news/article.php?id=5687.

8. K. Spiegel, R. Leproult, and E. Van Cauter, "Impact of Sleep
Debt on Metabolic and Endocrine Function," *Lancet* 354 (1999):
1,435–39.

9. M. Dallman, N. Pecoraro, S. Akano, S. LaFleur, F. Hourshyar
Gomez, M. Bell, S. Bhatnager, K. Laugero, and S. Manalo,
"Chronic Stress and Obesity: A New View of 'Comfort Food.' "
Proceedings of the National Academy of Sciences 100, no. 20 (Sep-
tember 30, 2003): 11, 696–701.

10. Hara Estroff Marano, "Chemistry and Craving," *Psychology Today*
(January/February 1993). Retrieved online May 25, 2007, from
http://psychologytoday.com/articles/index.php?term=pto-199301
01-000017&page=l.

7: Look Around: Hidden Cues That Make Us Eat

1. Brian Wansink and Jeffrey Sobal, "Mindless Eating: The 200
Daily Food Decisions We Overlook," *Environment and Behaviour*
39 (2007): 106–23.

2. Arthur Thompson and A. J. Strickland, *Strategic Management*,
11th edition (New York: McGraw-Hill, 1999).

3. Claire Caldwell and Sally A. Hibbert, "The Influence of Music
Tempo and Musical Preference on Restaurant Patrons' Behavior," *Psychology and Marketing* 19 (2002): 895–917.

4. Brian Wansink, "Environmental Factors That Increase the Food Intake and Consumption Volume of Unknowing Consumers," *Annual Review of Nutrition* 24, no. 1 (2004): 455.

5. Brian Wansink and Koert van Ittersum, "Bottoms Up! The Influence of Elongation on Pouring and Consumption Volume," *Journal of Consumer Research* 30 (December 2003).

6. Michael Tennesen, "Size Matters," *Better Health & Living* (2007). Retrieved online October 8, 2007, from http://www.better healthandliving.com/articles/size_matters/.

7. Mark Reutter, "Food Displays, Food Colors Affect How Much People Eat, Researcher Concludes," News Bureau, University of Illinois at Urbana–Champaign (May 10, 2004). Retrieved online October 10, 2007, from http://www.news.uiuc.edu/news/04/0510 food.html.

8. Barbara Rolls and Robert J. Barnett, *The Volumetrics Weight-Control Plan* (New York: HarperTorch, 2002).

9. Lisa Young and Marion Nestle, "The Contribution of Expanding Portion Sizes to the US Obesity Epidemic," *American Journal of Public Health* 92, no. 2 (February 2002).

10. Nancy DiMarco, "To Your Health: Hara Hachi Bu to You Too!" Texas Women's University. Retrieved online October 11, 2007, from http://www.twu.edu/twunews/your-health/hara.htm.

11. Science Daily, "Eating with Our Eyes: Why People Eat Less at Unbused Tables," Cornell University (April 11, 2007). Retrieved online December 15, 2007, from http://www.sciencedaily.com/ releases/2007/04/070409181631.htm.

12. B. Wansink, R. Kent, and S. Hoch, "An Anchoring and Adjustment Model of Purchase Quantity Decisions," *Journal of Marketing Research* 35, no. 1 (February 1998): 71–81.

13. Pierre Chandon and Brian Wansink, "Is Obesity Caused by Calorie Underestimation? A Psychophysical Model of Fast-Food Meal Size Estimation," *Journal of Marketing Research* 44, no. 1 (2007): 84–99.

8: Food, Marriage, and Family

1. N. Stroebele and J. de Castro, "Influence of Physiological and Subjective Arousal on Food Intake in Humans," *Nutrition* 22, no. 10: 996–1004.

9: Feasting on Emotions

1. J. Kleeberg, J. Boxer, E. J. Steiner, and G. J. Leeberg, "Studies on Almonds III. The Serotonin Content of Dried Sweet Almonds," *Archives internationales de pharmacodynamie et de thérapie* 2, no. 144 (August 2, 1963): 432–36.
2. Wansink, *Mindless Eating*, 144.
3. B. Lyman, "The Nutritional Values and Food Group Characteristics of Food Preferred During Various Emotions," *Journal of Psychology* 112 (1982): 121–27.
4. M. Macht, "Characteristics of Eating in Anger, Fear, Sadness, and Joy," *Appetite* 33 (1999): 65–71.
5. K. A. Patel and D. G. Schlundt, "Impact of Moods and Social Context on Eating Behavior," *Appetite* 36, no. 2 (2001): 111–18.
6. R. Kyung, J. Lumeng, D. Appugliese, N. Kaciroti, and R. Bradley, "Parenting Styles and Overweight Status in First Grade," *Pediatrics* 117, no. 6 (June 2006): 2047–54. Retrieved online August 8, 2007, from http://pediatrics.aappublications.org/cgi/content/abstract/117/6/2047.
7. H. Snoek, R. Engels, J. Janssens, and T. van Strien, "Parental Behaviour and Adolescents' Emotional Eating," *Appetite* 49, no. 1 (July 2007): 223–30.
8. D. Carmelli, G. E. Swan, and D. L. Bliwise, "Relationship of 30-Year Changes in Obesity to Sleep-Disordered Breathing in the Western Collaborative Group Study," *Obesity Research* 8, no. 9 (2000): 632–37.
9. R. Milligan, G. Waller, and B. Andrew, "Eating Disturbances in

Female Prisoners: The Role of Anger," *Eating Behaviors* 3, no. 2 (Summer 2002): 123–32.

10: The Power of Food Thoughts

1. Wansink, *Mindless Eating*, 79–80.
2. Karen Barrow, "Mindful Exercising: Thinking Your Body to Good Health?" Health Video (May 9, 2007). Retrieved online October 16, 2007, from http://4therapy.healthology.com/mental-health/ mental-health-news/article4239.htm.
3. G. Waller, V. Ohanian, C. Meyer, and S. Osman, "Cognitive Content among Bulimic Women: The Role of Core Beliefs," *International Journal of Eating Disorders* 28, no. 2 (September 2000): 235–41.
4. Science Daily, "Resistance to Thoughts of Chocolate Is Futile," University of Hertfordshire (October 29, 2007). Retrieved November 15, 2007, from http://www.sciencedaily.com/releases/ 2007/ten/071026213538.htm.
5. D. Wegner, D. Schneider, S. Carter, and T. White, "Paradoxical Effects of Thought Suppression," *Journal of Personality and Social Psychology* 53, no. 1 (July 1987): 5–13.

11: Spiritual Hunger Requires Spiritual Food

1. Science Daily, "Images of Desire: Brain Regions Activated by Food Craving Overlap with Areas Implicated in Drug Craving," Monell Chemical Senses Center (November 11, 2004). Retrieved April 18, 2008, from http://www.sciencedaily.com/ releases/2004/11/041108025155.htm.

12: Tackle Your Emotions

1. D. Tice, E. Bratslavsky, and R. Baumeister, "Emotional Distress Regulation Takes Precedence over Impulse Control: If You Feel Bad, Do It!" *Journal of Personality and Social Psychology* 30, no. 1 (2001): 53–66.
2. B. Bushman, R. Baumeister, and A. Stack, "Catharsis, Aggression and Persuasive Influence: Self-Fulfilling or Self-Defeating Prophecies?" *Journal of Personality and Social Psychology* 76, no. 3 (January 1999): 367–76.
3. "Sleep Hygiene: Helpful Hints to Help You Sleep," University of Maryland Sleep Disorders Center (2007). Retrieved online September 24, 2007, from http://www.umm.edu/sleep/sleep_hyg .html.

13: Renew Your Mind

1. C. S. Lewis, *The Case for Christianity* (New York: Touchstone Books, 1996).

14: Eating with People, Not Because of Them

1. John Gottman, "Why Marriages Fail," *The Family Therapy Networker* (May/June 1994): 41–48.

THE
Author, Book, & Conversation

DR. LINDA MINTLE, PH.D.

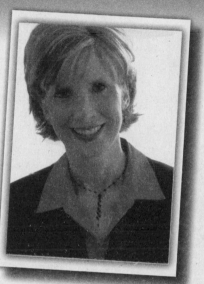

Known for her humor and practical advice, Dr. Linda, a national expert on marriage, family and eating issues, will motivate you toward positive life change. Her no-nonsense approach to everyday life and conversational style will inspire and uplift. For over twenty years, Dr. Linda has been in clinical practice as a licensed therapist, having worked in a variety of settings that have earned her several distinctions.

Dr. Mintle has authored thirteen books: *Raising Healthy Kids,* winner of the 2009 Mom's Choice Award, selected as book of the week by Dr. Laura and written for parents as a prevention to child obesity and overweight problems; *I Married You, Not Your Family*, a book aimed at strengthening marriage and preventing divorce endorsed by Dr. Laura; *Making Peace with Your Thighs*, a book aimed at helping women get off the scales and on with their lives; *Lose It for Life*, a bestseller coauthored with Stephen Arterburn that presents a total plan for losing weight and keeping it off; *A Daughter's Journey Home: Finding a Way to Love, Honor and Connect with Your Mother*, a book designed to help mothers and daughters develop more intimate connections; *Breaking Free*, a six-booklet series covering the topics of depression, anger and unwillingness to forgive, negative self-image, stress, anorexia and bulimia, and compulsive overeating; *Getting Unstuck*, a book that addresses the top three mental health issues for women; and *Kids Killing Kids*, a teen violence prevention book. Her newest release, *Press Pause Before You Eat*, a book that celebrates joyful eating and says good bye to mindless eating, will be available in spring 2009.

Married for thirty-four years and the mother of two teenagers, Dr. Linda currently resides in Virginia.

Why did you write *Press Pause Before You Eat?*

I wrote this book to change our relationship with food, to make eating something we enjoy, not something we do as we rush through our busy lives. Cultivating a life of mindfulness involves regulating what goes in your mouth for the right reasons. The concept of *press pause* is important to modern living. All of us need to slow down and think more about what we do and why we do it, especially when it comes to eating. Eating should be enjoyed, not a source of guilt or coping.

When did you, as a licensed therapist, first become interested in working with food and eating issues?

About thirty years ago, I helped develop one of the first eating disorder programs in the medical school where I was on the faculty. Our patients were mostly women who struggled with anorexia and bulimia. Over the years, more and more patients were coming to the institute for help with obesity and overeating. I began expanding my practice to include compulsive overeating and the psychological side of dealing with obesity and weight loss.

Why do so many of us have difficulty delaying gratification?

We live in a culture that reinforces impulsive behavior and does not teach self-control. Look around. We spend money we don't have, make decisions we regret, act out sexually, and basically do what feels good for the moment without much thought about the long-term consequences. Eating is no exception. The mistake is thinking that the answer to all this abundance and availability is willpower. Willpower doesn't win the impulsive battle. We need spiritual help here. Controlling our appetites requires more than human strength. It requires partnering with God and allowing His Spirit to empower us to make good choices.

You have a story in the book about a woman who used food to try and satisfy spiritual hunger. Do we often confuse the desire for food with spiritual emptiness?

Yes. We have an appetite for spiritual things that is often denied. There is a part of us that longs to be connected to something bigger than ourselves. This spiritual hunger can't be met through eating. Apart from God, we are restless. We were created to be satisfied by God. Until we develop an intimate relationship with Him, that spiritual hunger will persist.

248   Dr. Linda Mintle, Ph.D.
THE CONVERSATION   THE *Author, Book, & Conversation*
ABCs

STUDY QUESTIONS for *Press Pause Before You Eat*
Dr. Linda Mintle

1. When we are too busy to think about how and why we eat, we eat mindlessly. Learning to *pause* and slow down is an important part of eating better and with intention. Based on the information and suggestions in the book, what specific steps can you take to stop being so busy and take better care of yourself?

2. Review the signs of physical hunger. Each time you want to eat, go over those signs and decide if you are really hungry. If not, identify the cue or trigger that is prompting you to eat. For example, is it stress, an environmental cue, an emotion, a relationship issue, etc.? Keep the diary suggested in Chapters 5 and 8. Track your pat-terns of unintentional eating and notice what triggers you the most to eat when not hungry. Share with the group which type of cues trigger you the most.

3. Think about the meaning of food in your life. How does your cultural background influence your thoughts about food and eating? How do your family and your prior experiences with food play into how you use food today? Do you use food as a reward? Discuss these meanings in the group.

4. On a piece of paper, jot down the foods you tend to eat when you feel stressed. Now come up with strategies to de-stress yourself without using food. Make a list of things you can do when stress begins to mount in your life. Try substituting those things the next time you feel the urge to eat when stressed. Share your successes with the group.

5. Look at the eating area in your house, condo, or apartment. Does it look relaxing and inviting; do you even use it? Review all the environmental cues in Chapter 7 that make us overeat and check those against your own eating environment. What physical changes can you make to improve your eating area? Do you also need to commit to eating in that space and to taking more time with each meal? Finally, count the number of family meals eaten at the table. What can you do to increase that number? Have the group discuss the changes they made.

6. Evaluate the important relationships in your life. Are they meeting your expectations? Are your expectations realistic? Do you feel your intimacy needs are being met? Include your relationship with God in this evaluation. Now think about the times you may eat when upset or disappointed in these relationships. What can do you to resolve these issues other than use food to cope with negative feelings? Identify the relationships that lead you to eat without thinking. How often do you use prayer and time with God when you feel let down in relationships?

7. It is so difficult to make time to be quiet. Yet the Bible talks about the need for a pause to refresh our spirits. Look up these scriptures: Psalm 131:2; Psalm 130:5–6; Isaiah 30:15, 18; Psalm 40:1–3; Psalm 51:16. Read these scriptures and discuss the importance of waiting on the Lord.

8. This week, notice a time in which you are having food thoughts when you aren't hungry. Practice the skill of not resisting those thoughts but allowing them to come and go. Notice what happens to those thoughts. Write down your observations. Did this work better than trying to resist those thoughts? Did the craving pass? Practice this several times in the next week and report to the group on your experiences.

9. Take a few moments and examine your spiritual life. Do you practice spiritual disciplines or have you become complacent when it comes to spending time reading your Bible and sitting quietly before the Lord in prayer? If so, commit to those disciplines for the first time or once again. As you become more intimate with God, what do you notice about food cravings and mindless eating?

10. Eating in response to emotions is perhaps one of the most common things people do. Using the *press pause* principle, look at the chapter on regulating and tolerating emotions (Chapter 12) and come up with emotional rescues that would work. Decide which lifestyle changes you need to make and choose one to begin the process. Report on how it worked at the next study group.

11. Renewing the mind is a biblical concept that requires us to continually put on the mind of Christ. What can you do on a daily basis to fill your mind with truth and God's thought? Identify ways that will keep you operating in truth and empower your spirit with the fullness of God.

12. The final chapter in the book focuses on how to execute intentional eating. Evaluate each of the ten guidelines in terms of your own issues with food. Which of these will be the most difficult? Which of these is already a part of you? What can you do to keep these guidelines in place and develop a positive, healthy relationship with food? Discuss these in the group.